Sedation, Local and General Anesthesia in Dentistry

TANTE TANDPINE

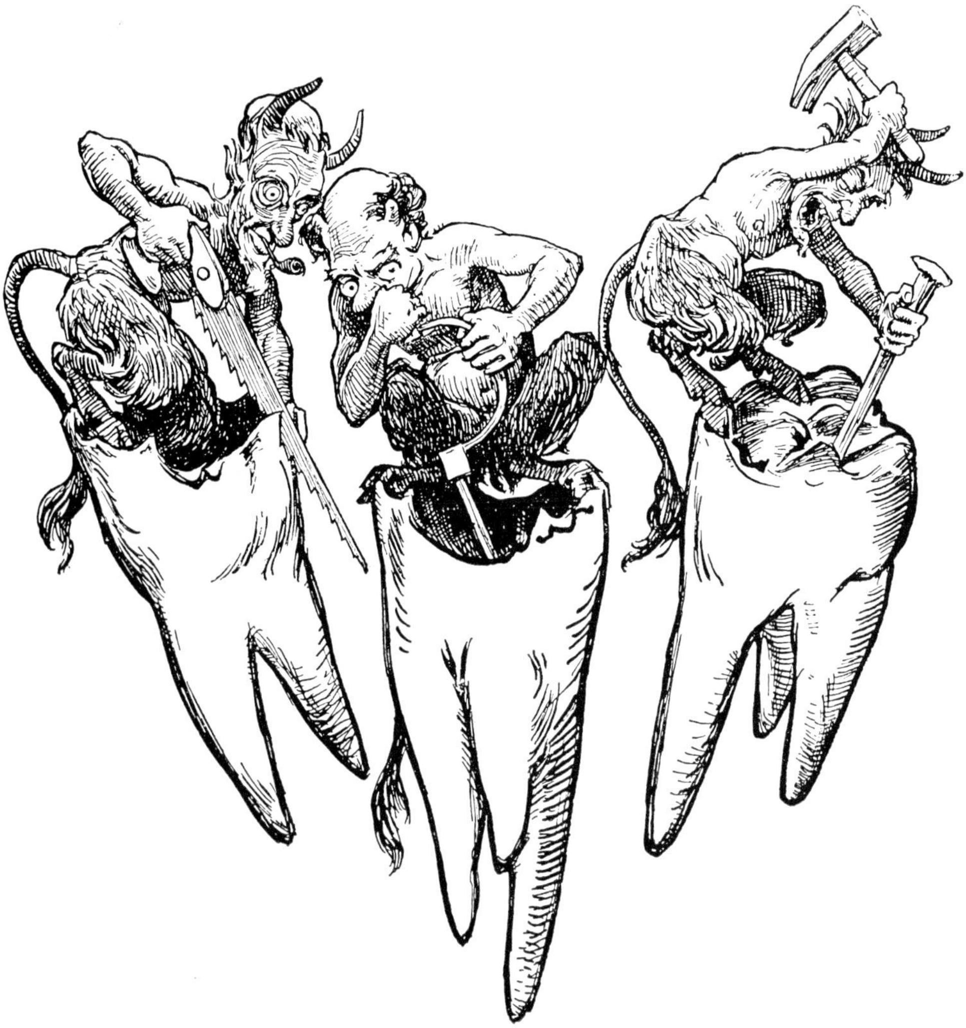

Hans Tegner's drawings for the tale of "Tante Tandpine" (Auntie Toothache) in the illustrated world edition of Hans Christian Andersen's *Fairy Tales* (1900) are among his best. Tegner (1853–1932) represents a toothache by three small imps attacking molars with saw, drill, and hammer and chisel; these vivacious imps symbolize what Andersen has to say about the Toothache Devil and Mrs. Toothache, Her Dreadfulness Satania Infernalis. Andersen wrote that the story originated with the first feelings of his youth. (Pindborg, J. J. and Marvitz, L.: *The Dentist in Art*, courtesy of Quadrangle Books, Inc., 1960.)

Sedation, Local and General Anesthesia in Dentistry

Niels Bjorn Jorgensen, D.D.S.
Emeritus Professor of Oral Surgery
Section on Anesthesia
School of Dentistry, Loma Linda University
Loma Linda, California

Jess Hayden, Jr., D.M.D., Ph.D.
Professor and Associate Dean, Coordinator for Research
College of Dentistry, University of Iowa
Iowa City, Iowa

Second Edition

Lea & Febiger · Philadelphia · 1972

ISBN 0-8121-0343-2

Published in Great Britain by Henry Kimpton Publishers, London

LIBRARY OF CONGRESS CATALOG CARD NUMBER 70:152026

Printed in the United States of America

Foreword

The technique of pain control associated with the name of Jorgensen and Loma Linda is recognized throughout the world. It provides control of patient anxiety together with safety, its major contribution to pain control being the concept of a titrated dose with an end-point dependent upon individual patient response. This end-point is reproducible, and is thus an excellent modality for the teaching of pain control; even the novice is able to judge dosage. Prior to my initiation of a detailed cardiorespiratory evaluation of the technique, I took the precaution of witnessing Dr. Jorgensen applying it in clinical practice. It is noteworthy that, not only was the clinical practice a success, but our research demonstrated that only minimal cardiorespiratory depression was produced. The technique has universal application for those dentists in practice who desire to alleviate pain and anxiety.

An avowed objective of the American Dental Society of Anesthesiology is to promote a total spectrum of pain control for the relief of anxiety in dental patients. The many techniques of analgesia in dentistry are considered in this book, and no one technique is suggested as a panacea. Significant attention is paid to anatomical detail with regard to innervation of the teeth, and the major role of local anesthesia in pain control in dentistry is recognized. Without satisfactory local anesthesia, analgesia can be achieved only with techniques which approximate general anesthesia. This attention to anatomical detail, with illustrations of anatomical dissections, and the discussion of local anesthetic technique highlight the fact that there is no substitute for the correctly placed needle tip for achieving local anesthesia. Most failures with local anesthetics are due to lack of anatomical knowledge.

Chapters of the book have been contributed by others active in the area of pain control in dentistry. In any program of analgesia and anesthesia, the dentist must be fully aware of the patient's physical status. Preoperative physical evaluation, which plays a vital role in the dentist's management of the patient and involves his skill as a doctor, is stressed, to be reemphasized in the psychic evaluation of the whole patient. The concept of team approach to pain control in dentistry is promoted as the only sensible way to overcome the problems of patient care in the office.

The proposed methodology and training program for the teaching of pain control provide guidance to those responsible for the training of future students. The endeavors of Dr. Jorgensen to promote pain control in dentistry have spanned the last five decades, beginning with the simple alcoholic draught and seen now in the refined inhalation and intravenous techniques. The reward for this effort is seen in the renewed interest of the dental profession in providing pain and anxiety-free dental treatment. The introduction of accurate inhalation-analgesia machines and more precise intravenous techniques should obviate the pitfalls of the past. Those of us involved in dental analgesia consider pain control an important feature of dental education. We are indebted to Dr. Jorgensen and his group for the part they have had in establishing the concepts of good patient care.

Gerald D. Allen
Associate Professor
Department of Anesthesiology
University of Washington School of Medicine

Preface

In the title of this second English edition of this text the word "sedation" is substituted for "premedication" because sedation more accurately describes the relief desired for a dental patient, whether obtained by inhalation, oral or parenteral routes. Further, wherever possible the word "sedation" has been used instead of "analgesia," because the word and state of analgesia have diverse connotations among practicing physicians and dentists, and use of the term may lead to undesirable misunderstandings.

During the several years since the publication of the first edition, it has been a pleasure to see arise a widespread recognition of, and a desire to control, the state of apprehension, fear and pain so often found among potential or actual dental patients. Since the manuscript for the second edition was written and submitted to the publishers, we have seen gratifyingly rewarded the efforts of a dedicated group of pain fighters. At the organizational level, the American Dental Society of Anesthesiology has formulated and gained acceptance for a position paper outlining and unifying the minimal requirements for the teaching of pain control in colleges of dentistry, and the National Institute of Dental Research has for the first time made the study of the cause of pain and its control in dental practice a definite and first-priority target.

We are pleased that the present climate of opinion makes advisable an expanded section on intravenous and inhalation sedation. At the same time we have buttressed the anatomical basis for venepuncture and the continued emphasis on local anesthesia. We still hold that local anesthesia is the basis of pain control in the general dental office. Although it is often regarded as too "simple" to require disciplined study, the science of obtaining routinely optimal local anesthesia is probably the least understood area of the dentist's armamentarium against pain.

Local anesthesia when preceded and accompanied by sedation with nitrous oxide and oxygen will effectively control pain and make possible routine treatment for many dental patients who, because of fear and lowered pain threshold, will either not seek dental care or else undergo an unnecessarily arduous treatment session.

We have ventured, with the encouragement and help of our contributors, to summarize our long-held and present convictions concerning the problems of dental pain control related to the delivery of dental treatment and the education of dental students. With some pride of editorship, we have noted a Spanish-language edition of the text. Essentially, however, this book is a continuing and enlarged expression of the philosophy of the control of pain associated with dental treatment as taught at Loma Linda University since the mid 1940s. To our contributors and colleagues—basic health scientists, dentists and physicians from our respective universities and elsewhere—who have so willingly helped us with these two editions, and to others who have farsightedly and tenaciously fought for the elimination of apprehension, anxiety and pain in dental practice, we express our continuing gratitude.

North Hollywood, California N.B.J.

Iowa City, Iowa J.H., Jr.

Acknowledgments

As the second edition of the text is distributed we again wish to thank our fellow contributors and our colleagues in the university community for their willingness to give of their time and support. Most of the illustrations were seen in the first edition, and Mrs. Beverly Sandquist, R.N., Mrs. Irene Cathey, Miss Judith Lipsett, and Mrs. Janet E. Mogill deserve special recognition for their repeated sittings for the photographing of the various injections. Most of the photographs are products of the perseverance and artistic skill of Messrs. Edward N. Hamilton and E. Jones. Mrs. Lucille Innes and Mr. George Buckley lent their talents to the clarification of the photographs through drawings, labeling, and the preparation of legends, and to what we believe are clear and helpful illustrations of regional anatomy. Professor W. K. Metcalf kindly reviewed the chapter on anatomy from serial gross sections through the final typing. Our friends and colleagues from overseas, namely Drs. Henning Ruben, S. L. Drummond-Jackson, D. H. Tompsett and J. Pindborg, have made available facts, figures and illustrations. To our cooperative typists, Mmes. Pat Dubler, Jan Morgan, Barbara Huff and Marian Van Fossen, our thanks and appreciation.

N.B.J.
J.H., Jr.

Contributors

Evans, Harrison S., M.D.
Professor and Chairman, Department of Psychiatry, Schools of Medicine and Dentistry, Loma Linda University

Hubbell, Adrian O., D.D.S.
Private practice of oral surgery, Long Beach, California. Former Special Lecturer in Anesthesia, Postgraduate Instruction Divisions of Georgetown and Tufts Universities

McCarthy, Frank M., M.D., D.D.S.
Clinical Professor, Oral Surgery, University of Southern California School of Dentistry; Director, University of Southern California Anesthesia Service, Dental Section, Los Angeles County Hospital

Mitchell, Clifford L., Ph.D.
Professor of Pharmacology, College of Medicine, University of Iowa

Royer, R. Quentin, D.D.S., M.S.
Private practice of oral surgery, Long Beach, California. Clinical Professor, Oral Surgery, University of Southern California, Los Angeles

Contents

Section I

Patient Evaluation

Chapter 1

Physical Evaluation

Frank M. McCarthy, M.D., D.D.S., M.S.

Physical evaluation before dental therapy is mandatory. No longer is the question "Are you in good health?" sufficient. The dental practitioner is morally and legally obligated to perform a reasonable screening procedure in order to protect the health and safety of every patient.

Death, serious illness, and minor reactions may be directly related to dental anesthesia or treatment. Such complications, while not always preventable, can frequently be minimized or avoided by proper pretreatment evaluation.

The desirability of routine dental physical evaluation has heightened in recent years because of lengthening dental appointments with an attendant increase in physical and emotional stress. Further adding to the necessity for proper physical evaluation are sophisticated psychosedation techniques and the increasing number of patients of geriatric age.

The dentist's goal in evaluation is simply to determine the physical and emotional ability of a particular patient to tolerate a specific dental procedure. The goal is not to diagnose or treat the medical problem, although reasonably accurate diagnoses will be achieved by the use of a proper evaluation technique and by experience. We, as dentists, wish to produce an evaluation factor by which it is determined whether we may proceed with dental treatment in relative safety or whether medical consultation is indicated prior to dental treatment.

The function of the physician is to reach a diagnosis and to treat the medical problem. When any doubt exists regarding the medical status of the dentist's patient, the patient's physician should be consulted. The physician is a vital member of the health team, and will be more than willing to discuss the dental treatment plans as they relate to the specific medical problems of the patient. The dentist has a responsibility to the patient to consult the physician and to be guided but not directed by his advice. In regard to the dental treatment the final responsibility to the patient is the dentist's, and cannot be equally shared by the physician except under unusual circumstances. The physician's advice should be received with an open mind and the dental treatment plan with the anticipated problems discussed with the physician.

In most cases, consultation with the physician will result in little alteration of the dental treatment plan. In some cases the plan may be markedly altered, and in rare instances it may be necessary to delay treatment or postpone it indefinitely. It makes little sense to rehabilitate dentally a patient with terminal cancer, nor does it make sense to subject a high-risk cardiac patient to prolonged, stress-producing restorative dentistry. The dentist must be prepared to justify anything except emergency dental treatment for the high-risk patient.

The evaluation technique described here is designed to be used by all dentists, regardless of their past training or experience. The general practitioner may utilize one of the standard histories only. As experience is gained, and particularly if he supplements his knowledge with continuing education, the dentist will progress further into full evaluation of the patient. Depending on his background and interest in the subject, the general practitioner may readily develop the ability to make a detailed and highly accurate judgment of his patient's physical status.

The standard histories which follow can be used by all dentists, irrespective of their type of practice. The oral surgeon is obligated to make a detailed analysis, particularly when general anesthesia is to be used; yet the general practitioner should not feel that he is excused from the obligation of evaluation. The risk of local anesthesia or any dental treatment in a particular case may be very high, as mortality statistics in the general dental office will bear out.

PRELIMINARY HISTORY

Every patient in the dental office should be required to complete a standard medical history. Two forms which I recommend are taken from the 1971–72 edition of *Accepted Dental Therapeutics*, American Dental Association.

The short-form ADT medical history (Fig. 1–1) is adequate for the experienced practitioner and it produces a reliable risk factor. It was originally conceived by the Anesthesia Service, Dental Section, Los Angeles County/University of Southern California Medical Center for use prior to outpatient general anesthesia, and it has been modified to apply equally well to all dental therapy with or without psychosedation or general anesthesia.

The long-form ADT medical history (Fig. 1–2) is recommended for the inexperienced practitioner. It is an excellent teaching aid and can serve as a departure point for complete physical diagnosis.

Other routine medical history forms in general use are equally applicable; the choice rests with the practitioner.

The new patient completes the history and standard form in the reception room, after which the dental assistant reviews the medical record with the patient to make certain that the form is complete. The patient and the assistant sign the dated form, thereby providing evidence that the history was taken and is accurate.

When the patient is met in consultation, the dentist briefly reviews the form himself and proceeds with evaluation as indicated. When the patient returns to the office after a period of time, it is my custom to have the assistant ask the patient if he has had any health problems or is taking any medication not previously recorded or discussed. Appropriate notation is made on the record and initialed by the assistant. A new health history is not necessary.

FOLLOW-UP HISTORY

The detailed or follow-up history is obtained by the dentist after reviewing the preliminary history form. This includes further specific evaluation of positive information obtained by means of the preliminary questions. In most cases, little time is spent on this portion of the evaluation. If the preliminary history discloses points for

HEALTH QUESTIONNAIRE

Date____________________

Name______________________________Address________________________
Last First Middle Number & Street

____
City State Zip Code Home & Business Phone

Age______Sex______Height______Weight______Occupation____________

Married______Spouse____________________________Single______

Closest Relative____________________________Phone____________

If you are completing this form for another person, what is your relationship to that person?

PLEASE ANSWER EACH QUESTION	Check One Yes	No
1. Have you been a patient in a hospital during the past 2 years?..................	☐	☐
2. Have you been under the care of a physician during the past 2 years?...........	☐	☐
3. Have you taken any kind of medicine or drugs during the past year?.............	☐	☐
4. Are you allergic to penicillin or any drugs or medicine?.........................	☐	☐
5. Have you ever had any excessive bleeding requiring special treatment?........	☐	☐

6. Circle any of the following which you have had:

heart trouble	asthma	arthritis
congenital heart lesions	cough	stroke
heart murmur	diabetes	epilepsy
high blood pressure	tuberculosis	psychiatric treatment
anemia	hepatitis	sinus trouble
rheumatic fever	jaundice	

	Yes	No
7. (Women) Are you pregnant now?..	☐	☐
8. Have you had any other serious illnesses?......................................	☐	☐

TO BE ANSWERED ONLY BY PATIENTS RECEIVING SEDATION OR GENERAL ANESTHESIA

	Yes	No
9. Have you had anything to eat or drink within the last 4 hours?..................	☐	☐
10. Are you wearing a removable dental appliance?................................	☐	☐
11. Are you wearing contact lenses?..	☐	☐

12. Who is to drive you home today?

a. Name____________________________________

Reviewed by__________________ Signature__________________

FIG. 1–1. Short-form medical history, from *Accepted Dental Therapeutics*, American Dental Association, 1971–72. This form produces a reliable risk factor and is adequate for the experienced practitioner. It applies equally well to all dental therapy.

HEALTH QUESTIONNAIRE

Date__________

Name__________ Address__________
Last First Middle Number & Street

____
City State Zip Code Home & Business Phone

Age____ Sex____ Height____ Weight____ Occupation________

Married____ Spouse__________ Single____

Closest Relative__________ Phone________

If you are completing this form for another person, what is your relationship to that person.

____

In the following questions, circle yes or no, whichever applies. Your answers are for our records only and will be considered confidential.

1. Has there been any change in your general health within the past year........... YES NO
2. My last physical examination was on__________
3. Are you now under the care of a physician.. YES NO
   a. If so, what is the condition being treated__________
4. The name and address of my physician is__________
   ____
   ____
5. Have you had any serious illness or operation.................................... YES NO
   a. If so, what was the illness or operation__________
6. Have you been hospitalized or had a serious illness within the past five (5) years... YES NO
   a. If so, what was the problem__________
7. Do you have or have you had any of the following diseases or problems.
   a. Rheumatic fever or rheumatic heart disease.................................. YES NO
   b. Congenital heart lesions... YES NO
   c. Cardiovascular disease (heart trouble, heart attack, coronary insufficiency, coronary occlusion, high blood pressure, arteriosclerosis, stroke)............. YES NO
      1) Do you have pain in chest upon exertion................................... YES NO
      2) Are you ever short of breath after mild exercise............................ YES NO
      3) Do your ankles swell.. YES NO
      4) Do you get short of breath when you lie down, or do you require extra pillows when you sleep.. YES NO
   d. Allergy.. YES NO
   e. Sinus trouble.. YES NO
   f. Asthma or hay fever... YES NO
   g. Hives or a skin rash.. YES NO
   h. Fainting spells or seizures.. YES NO
   i. Diabetes... YES NO
      1) Do you have to urinate (pass water) more than six times a day............. YES NO
      2) Are you thirsty much of the time.. YES NO
      3) Does your mouth frequently become dry................................... YES NO
   j. Hepatitis, jaundice or liver disease... YES NO
   k. Arthritis.. YES NO
   l. Inflammatory rheumatism (painful swollen joints)............................ YES NO
   m. Stomach ulcers.. YES NO
   n. Kidney trouble... YES NO
   o. Tuberculosis... YES NO
   p. Do you have a persistent cough or cough up blood............................ YES NO
   q. Low blood pressure.. YES NO
   r. Venereal disease.. YES NO
   s. Other__________

FIG. 1–2. Long-form medical history, from *Accepted Dental Therapeutics*, American Dental Association, 1971–72. This form is an excellent teaching aid and can serve as a departure point for complete physical diagnosis. It is recommended for the inexperienced practitioner.

8. Have you had abnormal bleeding associated with previous extractions, surgery, or trauma .... YES NO
   a. Do you bruise easily .... YES NO
   b. Have you ever required a blood transfusion .... YES NO

   If so, explain the circumstances ____________________

9. Do you have any blood disorder such as anemia .... YES NO
10. Have you had surgery or x-ray treatment for a tumor, growth, or other condition of your mouth or lips .... YES NO
11. Are you taking any drug or medicine .... YES NO

    If so, what ____________________
12. Are you taking any of the following:
    a. Antibiotics or sulfa drugs .... YES NO
    b. Anticoagulants (blood thinners) .... YES NO
    c. Medicine for high blood pressure .... YES NO
    d. Cortisone (steroids) .... YES NO
    e. Tranquilizers .... YES NO
    f. Antihistamines .... YES NO
    g. Aspirin .... YES NO
    h. Insulin, tolbutamide (Orinase) or similar drug .... YES NO
    i. Digitalis or drugs for heart trouble .... YES NO
    j. Nitroglycerin .... YES NO

    k. Other ____________________
13. Are you allergic or have you reacted adversely to:
    a. Local anesthetics .... YES NO
    b. Penicillin or other antibiotics .... YES NO
    c. Sulfa drugs .... YES NO
    d. Barbiturates, sedatives, or sleeping pills .... YES NO
    e. Aspirin .... YES NO
    f. Iodine .... YES NO

    g. Other ____________________
14. Have you had any serious trouble associated with any previous dental treatment .... YES NO

    If so, explain ____________________

15. Do you have any disease, condition, or problem not listed above that you think I should know about .... YES NO

    If so, please explain ____________________

16. Are you employed in any situation which exposes you regularly to x-rays or other ionizing radiation .... YES NO
17. Are you wearing contact lenses .... YES NO

WOMEN

18. Are you pregnant .... YES NO
19. Do you have any problems associated with your menstrual period .... YES NO

Remarks:

____
SIGNATURE OF PATIENT

____
SIGNATURE OF DENTIST

FIG. 1–2. *Continued.*

further investigation, and the dentist is unable or unwilling to proceed further without consultation, a conference with the patient's physician is arranged at this time.

To assist in continuing with a detailed history, certain broad categories of disease will now be reviewed, and questions will be suggested for evaluation of the diseases in respect to dentistry. Only the most common high-risk diseases will be covered. I have also granted myself a certain license for the purpose of discussing the medical background of each disease entity.

METABOLIC DISEASES

Diabetes Mellitus

Do not treat the uncontrolled diabetic. His health picture makes him a poor candidate for withstanding dental stress, and it has been shown that emotional stress increases glycemia and the tendency to diabetic acidosis and coma.

Most diabetics can give an accurate estimate of their current status, since they routinely test their urine for sugar. If reaction to the urine test is negative or there is a trace of or a 1+ reaction for sugar, little problem with dental treatment would be expected. If the patient is doubtful regarding the control of his diabetes, question him regarding abnormal thirst, abnormal urine output, and abnormal weight loss. The presence of any or all of these symptoms constitutes a sign of uncontrolled diabetes. If doubt exists, a medical consultation is in order. It should be noted that, in the severe diabetic, control cannot readily be obtained by use of such insulin substitutes as oral Diabinese. If the patient is taking one of the oral hypoglycemic agents or the disease is controlled by diet alone, it may be assumed that the diabetes is not severe.

There is a marked tendency toward early development of arteriosclerosis in the diabetic, whether the diabetes is controlled or not. In evaluating the diabetic it is well to inquire into possible symptoms of heart failure and angina pectoris.

Frequently the meal before a dental appointment is inadequate or is missed entirely due to apprehension, and in these days of quadrant dentistry it is common for the patient to miss another meal or even two after the appointment. If the contemplated dental procedure may result in the missing of several meals, I direct the patient to decrease his normal insulin by half on the day of treatment in order to prevent the possibility of insulin shock. An elevated blood sugar level for a short period is harmless.

Hyperthyroidism

For our purposes a history of hyperthyroidism should suggest the possibility of heart disease and angina pectoris. In addition, the patient with moderately severe hyperthyroidism suffers from tachycardia, sweating, headache, and nervous manifestations which make him a poor candidate for usual dental care.

Adrenal Insufficiency

The possibility of adrenal insufficiency may be assumed in a patient who has taken an adrenocortical agent (cortisone, hydrocortisone, etc.) within the preceding six months. Irreversible shock may occur with such minor stress as that instigated by a local anesthetic injection or a simple dental extraction. The patient's physician should be consulted and in all probability he will reinstitute the adrenocortical therapy prior to dental treatment.

CARDIOVASCULAR AND CEREBROVASCULAR DISEASE

Heart Failure

Known more precisely as cardiac decompensation or congestive heart failure, a failing heart represents one of the most common risks in a patient treated in the dental office. For purposes of understanding, I have included both right- and left-sided heart failure in this classification, although they normally are discussed separately.

The main symptom of heart failure is dyspnea, or shortness of breath; the second most important symptom is edema, which starts in the ankles. For the dentist's purposes, evaluation by degree of dyspnea is relatively accurate.

The following are questions recommended for the evaluation of heart failure:

1. Can you carry on your usual normal activities without shortness of breath or undue fatigue?

COMMENT: An affirmative answer represents a good risk if other points are negative. No point in evaluation is more important than the fact that the functional capacity of the patient allows him to carry on normal activities.

2. Can you climb a flight of stairs without resting?

COMMENT: If the answer is affirmative the patient is a good risk if other points are negative.

3. Do your ankles swell as the day progresses?

COMMENT: Swelling of the ankles is a compensatory mechanism in chronic right-sided heart failure.

4. Have you ever awakened at night with shortness of breath?

COMMENT: Shortness of breath occurring at night is known as paroxysmal nocturnal dyspnea, a serious symptom; it is the result of acute failure with pulmonary edema. Consultation with the physician is advised.

5. Must you remain in a sitting position in order to breathe comfortably?

COMMENT: The inability to breathe except in the upright position is known as orthopnea—a serious symptom; it is a compensatory mechanism to confine pulmonary edema to the lung bases and to keep ventilatory capacity at a maximum. Consultation is recommended.

6. How many pillows do you use to facilitate breathing comfort while sleeping?

COMMENT: If two or three pillows are used, the presence of orthopnea is indicated.

7. Have you had a recent large increase in weight?

COMMENT: Marked weight gain may indicate rapid fluid accumulation and onset of acute failure. The patient will have swollen ankles and legs and possibly a distended abdomen. Consultation is recommended.

8. Are you taking medication?

COMMENT: If the patient is taking a diuretic, chronic heart failure should be suspected. If he is taking digitalis or a digitalis glycoside (digoxin, digitoxin, Lanoxin, etc.), it may be assumed that the patient has had or is having an episode of heart failure. If the patient has resumed normal activities since digitalization, and other points are negative, the failure is compensated and the patient is a good risk.

The following functional reserve classification is an aid in determining the current cardiovascular status in cardiac failure cases and is of assistance in planning dental treatment. This classification is also helpful when there is a history of pulmonary disease such as lung abscess, tuberculosis, emphysema, bronchial asthma, and bronchiectasis.

Functional Reserve Classification (McCarthy)

Class 1. No dyspnea with normal exertion.

Class 2. Mild dyspnea with exertion; may rest at the top of a flight of stairs.

COMMENT: Assuming that other points are negative, patients in Class 1 or 2 represent good risks for all dental treatment. If the Class 2 patient is quite apprehensive, sedation to reduce emotional and physical stress should be considered.

Class 3. Dyspnea with normal activities; comfortable at rest in any position; may have a tendency toward orthopnea, and may have a history of paroxysmal nocturnal dyspnea; rests before reaching the top of a flight of stairs.

COMMENT: This patient represents a definite risk; consultation is recommended. Sedation during dental treatment is strongly recommended. Appointments should be short; treatment should not be carried to the limit of tolerance.

Class 4. Dyspnea and orthopnea at all times. The patient will rest on numerous occasions when climbing a flight of stairs, if he is able to negotiate them at all.

COMMENT: Such a patient represents a serious risk; only emergency dental treatment should be considered. The patient's physician should be in attendance if possible, or at least within call.

Angina Pectoris

Angina pectoris is also known as "paroxysmal cardiac pain" and as "anginal syndrome." A patient with angina pectoris represents a considerably greater risk than does the average patient having heart failure. The mortality rate in a patient with angina is at least 30 per cent higher than in the average subject. It must be remembered that the attack can become irreversible, proceeding to coronary thrombosis and possibly to death.

The patient will give a history of recurrent attacks of substernal pain, varying from mild to severe. There is often radiation of pain to the left shoulder or arm, infrequently to the right shoulder and back. The pain often is precipitated by exertion or excitement, and usually is relieved by rest. The patient has usually taken nitroglycerin for relief of pain. Consultation with the patient's physician regarding the planned dental treatment is desirable.

Recommended Handling of the Anginal Patient

1. Routine sedation is strongly advised. These patients do not tolerate emotional stress well.
2. Make every effort to achieve effective local anesthesia; use the proper technique.
3. Premedicate with nitroglycerin sublingually about five minutes before administering the local anesthetic. Use the patient's supply of nitroglycerin if possible. A significant number of anginal patients (estimated at up to 10 per cent) will exhibit a paradoxical reaction to nitroglycerin when taken in a dosage higher than they normally find effective, and an anginal attack will ensue. If the patient is not carrying his usual supply, use nitroglycerin in the dosage of 1/200 grain. I do not recommend that the commonly used higher dosage forms of 1/150 and 1/100 grain be stocked.
4. For the relief of mild anginal pain during dental treatment, give one or two 1/200 grain tablets of nitroglycerin sublingually. One need not fear a paradoxical reaction when the anginal syndrome already exists. For rapid relief of severe anginal pain, have the patient inhale the contents of an amyl nitrite ampule.
5. Keep the procedure as short as possible, and make every effort to avoid reaching the limit of tolerance.
6. Remember that the average anginal patient's risk level is about the same as that of the cardiac patient in Class 3 functional reserve.
7. If the patient has almost daily episodes of chest pain, especially associated with meals and/or emotional stress, consider him a serious risk. Emergency dental treatment only is recommended.

Coronary Thrombosis

Coronary thrombosis is also known as heart attack, coronary occlusion and, more properly, myocardial infarction. This patient, as does the one with angina, represents a mortality risk at least 30 per cent greater than does the average patient.

At onset, symptoms of coronary thrombosis are similar to those of angina pectoris but the substernal pain is not relieved by nitrites or rest, and dyspnea, weakness, and sweating are common.

Most postcoronary patients know the proper diagnosis of their condition. If they are not aware of the nature of their heart trouble, its basis can easily be established by reviewing the history. There usually will be a history of hospitalization followed by some weeks or months of inactivity at home. Consultation with the physician is desirable prior to treatment planning.

Recommended Handling of the Postcoronary Patient

Routine office handling of the postcoronary patient exactly duplicates the routine handling of the anginal patient, with three exceptions:

1. Routine premedication with nitroglycerin is open to debate, and therefore is not recommended. However, it is definitely recommended if the patient has current episodes of angina pectoris. Dosage forms are the same as in angina.
2. Do not perform any elective dental treatment for the postcoronary patient for at least six months after the attack. It takes that long for the lesion to heal and the cardiac function to become stabilized.
3. If the patient is taking an anticoagulant (heparin, Dicumarol, Coumadin, Hedulin, etc.), and most postcoronary patients do so for at least a year after the attack, dental treatment during which even mild bleeding may occur should be avoided until the patient's status has been discussed with the physician.

Hypertension

When the preliminary medical form shows a history of hypertension, the possible existence of heart failure and angina pectoris should be investigated. It is natural to think of stroke first when confronted with a hypertensive history, but the fact is that 65 per cent of hypertensives die of heart disease, whereas only 20 per cent demonstrate predominantly cerebral symptoms.

When taking the follow-up history, inquiry should be made to determine if the patient has ever had transient episodes of syncope, speech defects, or paresthesia or paralysis of an extremity. These temporary episodes do not constitute a true stroke, but are prodromal only and usually represent temporary cerebral insufficiency. A patient with such a history should be handled in the office as if he had had an actual stroke.

The detailed history may disclose the fact that the patient had an actual stroke in the past (cerebrovascular accident [CVA], cerebral apoplexy, cerebral hemorrhage, cerebral thrombosis). This would have been marked, by order of onset, as follows: intense headache; vomiting; drowsiness; possible coma or convulsions; paralysis, with or without recovery.

Recommended Handling of the Post-CVA Patient

1. A medical consultation is desirable if the patient's physical status is doubtful.
2. No elective dental treatment should be given for at least six months after the episode.
3. Keep appointments short.
4. Sedation is highly desirable, but should be used with great care and should not be carried to the point that the patient experiences extreme drowsiness or depression. Heavy sedation depresses cerebral circulation and can initiate cerebral thrombosis.

PHYSICAL EXAMINATION

The standard history form, plus the indicated follow-up inquiries, will, in most cases, provide an adequate physical evaluation in dentistry. However, no physical evaluation is complete without a physical examination.

Inspection

Inspection of the patient represents the first step of every physical examination. The dentist has been doing this, perhaps without realizing it, since he started practice.

The dentist should train himself actually to see the patient when checking the preliminary history or taking a follow-up history. Several points to observe are:

1. The color of the skin:
   - Cyanosis—heart disease
   - Pallor—anemia, fear, tendency toward syncope
   - Flushing—fever, atropine overdosage, apprehension, hyperthyroidism
   - Jaundice—liver disease
2. The eyes:
   - Exophthalmos—hyperthyroidism
3. The conjunctiva:

Pallor—anemia
Jaundice—liver disease

4. The hands:
   Tremor — hyperthyroidism, apprehension, hysteria, paralysis agitans, epilepsy, multiple sclerosis, senility
5. The fingers:
   Clubbing—cardiopulmonary disease
   Cyanosis of nail beds—heart disease
6. The neck:
   Jugular vein distension—right-sided heart failure
7. The ankles:
   Swelling—varicose veins, right-sided heart failure, kidney disease
8. The respiratory rate, particularly with heart failure:
   Normal for adult—16 to 18 per minute
   Normal for child—24 to 28 per minute

Blood Pressure and Pulse

In addition to the usual inspection, I feel that determination of the blood pressure in all patients over six years of age should become routine in the dental office, and that the blood pressure should be redetermined when the patient has not been examined for a period of six months or longer.

Taking the blood pressure is mandatory if psychosedation is planned, and both pulse and blood pressure should be determined in cases of suspected cardiovascular or cerebrovascular disease.

Pulse Consideration

1. Pulse rate varies from 60 to 80 per minute in the normal adult, 80 to 100 per minute in the normal child.

COMMENT: A rate of less than 60 or more than 110 in the adult should be viewed with suspicion, and may be sufficient evidence to justify a medical consultation.

2. The pulse rate should be within normal limits and should be both strong and regular.
3. Any irregularity of the pulse, other than a very occasional premature contraction (extrasystole, dropped beat), is an indication for medical consultation.

EXAMPLES:

(*a*) Complete irregularity of the pulse (complete arrhythmia, pulsus irregularis perpetuus) usually indicates atrial fibrillation; this may or may not be serious in respect to dental treatment.

(*b*) Pulsus alternans, which is regular alternation in the size or strength of the pulsations, indicates severe myocardial damage.

Blood Pressure

The dental assistant may be easily trained to take the patient's blood pressure as a matter of routine, although I find it wise to check the reading personally if it is abnormal.

One will be gratified by the number of undiagnosed and often asymptomatic cases of hypertension which this routine measure will disclose. Patients will be most appreciative of this health service, but, more important, alertness on the dentist's part can result in the early and effective medical treatment of hypertension, and the dentist's own treatment plan may well be altered by the discovery.

The blood pressure may vary from 90/60 to 150/100 mm Hg in the normal adult. Since it may vary as much as 20 to 30 mm over a short period because of exertion or anxiety, several readings should be made when abnormal values are obtained, and it should be assumed that the lowest reading is the correct one for the patient.

There is no simple way of estimating by blood pressure readings alone whether the patient's hypertension is mild or severe. The evaluation must depend on the blood pressure reading and, more important, on the overall evaluation of the patient. A patient who is taking an antihypertensive drug, who has a history of a stroke and a blood pressure of 160/100 may be a far greater risk in the dental office than a patient with untreated essential hypertension, a reading of 190/120, and a total lack of symptoms referable to hypertension. If any doubt exists regarding the propriety of treatment, the patient's physician should be consulted.

Breath-Holding Test

At the completion of history taking and physical examination, there may still be serious doubts about the functional reserve of a patient with cardiovascular or pulmonary disease. If so, the breath-holding test is very helpful, and it is extremely accurate. It serves as an office flight-of-stairs test.

Technique

1. The patient takes a deep breath.
2. The patient pinches his nostrils together in order to prevent exhalation and also breathing through his nose.
3. The patient holds his breath for as long as possible, while the dentist times the interval.

Interpretation

1. The upper limits vary greatly and may be more than 35 to 45 seconds.
2. A test result of 15 seconds or less should be viewed with suspicion, especially if there is evidence of cardiovascular or respiratory disease.

Laboratory Tests

For years, prior to general anesthesia, hospitalized patients have had a minimum laboratory examination consisting of a routine urinalysis and a complete blood count. In the offices of most oral surgeons such examinations have never become routine, although in a small minority a hemoglobin determination and a check of the urine for sugar are made. It is doubtful if such examinations add significantly to the usual dental evaluation outlined here.

If the dentist has doubts regarding possible kidney disease, anemia, bleeding tendencies, diabetes, etc., I feel that it would be wise to refer the patient to a clinical laboratory, depending on the dentist's background and experience in interpreting such tests, or to the patient's physician for appropriate examination, tests, and opinion.

Chapter

2

Psychological Aspects of Dental Practice

Harrison S. Evans, M.D.

The doctor's interest and concern for his patient should extend beyond the limits of his particular medical specialty. His breadth of interest and concern is part of what distinguishes him from the technician trained to understand and deal with a part without being knowledgeable or informed about the larger whole. A technician may be expected to have great procedural skill, but he is not expected to be a person of medical depth or breadth.

On the other hand, the doctor, whether a dentist, proctologist, urologist, ophthalmologist, etc., is expected to understand that medical problems, even though circumscribed, are more than of local significance—that the whole person is involved in different ways and at different levels.

In this section on psychological aspects of dental practice we are going to consider the way in which the whole person is involved in his illness. What does the patient's dental problem and its treatment mean to him? What are his feelings about it and how is his reaction influenced by the meaning and feelings? This dimension of dental practice should not be ignored or considered unimportant. Good professional care requires not only technical knowledge and skill but also an interest in and a concern for the patient as a person, with an understanding of his feelings and emotional needs.

It is recognized that the successful dentist (or physician) intuitively understands his patient's feelings and attitudes, and instinctively cares for them while attending to the medical problem. This innate capacity to understand and to react intuitively is an invaluable asset to the clinician. However, it is both unwise and now unnecessary to depend upon one's intuitive faculties alone.

There has accumulated over the years a body of scientific knowledge about people and personality which can be taught and acquired, thereby enriching and augmenting the doctor's natural talents for understanding. In terms of total patient care—comfort and successful and satisfying treatment—this body of knowledge is not of secondary importance to a knowledge of anatomy, physiology, or surgery. In this chapter, some of this accumulated knowledge and understanding of people will be presented.

HOLISM

An understanding and acceptance of the concept of holism can contribute to the depth and breadth of patient care. It conveys the idea that each patient must be seen as a whole, and not just in terms of his parts.

When we refer to the "whole" we are speaking of the patient as a person, as a unique personality, with his own set of hopes, fears, feelings and values. When we see our patient holistically we do not see his parts as something existing and functioning in isolation apart from him as a person, which indeed they do not. They are meaningful and significant parts of him, and contribute to his total being. It is important to realize that what he contemplates about anticipated changes or losses of his parts can add to or diminish his sense of wholeness. This fact must be taken into consideration as physical, dental or medical procedures are planned.

In this holistic frame of reference, every doctor's task, then, is to keep in mind a patient's personality, where the patient's sense of wholeness exists on the basis of meaning and significance. At the personality level every change has meaning. Attention to and support of the patient's personality through preserving and maintaining as much as possible of what is psychologically important to him represents the highest type of professional care. When drastic but essential changes are medically indicated, it is part of a doctor's task to assist the patient in adapting to these changes so that the integrity of the personality can be maintained.

FEAR VERSUS ANXIETY

Fear and anxiety are emotional reactions elaborated by the personality and based upon meaning and significance. A situation may arouse fear or anxiety because it signifies danger or threat to the person, even though in reality danger may not exist; the danger is not precisely the situation itself, but the way in which a person sees the situation and what it means to him. Nevertheless, certain basic life situations are prone to arouse anxiety in almost anyone, and among them is going to the dentist or physician.

Fear, as compared with anxiety, can be considered in general a realistic emotional response. It is a reaction to a concrete situation constituting an actual danger or threat to the person's well-being. For example, every person would experience fear if he were subjected to war combat or if, as a mountain climber, he were inching his way over vertical mountainside. Anxiety, on the other hand, is the response to situations that are dangerous only symbolically. Anxiety, in contrast to fear, is intangible. It is a vague apprehension which serves to alert the organism to possible dangers that are not clearly defined.

We understand anxiety as having its roots in childhood. The child is small, weak and vulnerable, and at this time everything seems potentially threatening. However, with growth and experience one learns that everything is not dangerous; one gradually develops confidence and trust in others and in one's self. Anxiety largely apparently disappears, but it lies latent within a person's unconscious memory. New situations reminiscent of former dangers can easily arouse old anxieties to color the new situation with dangers that may not actually be present except in the imagination.

Anxiety, even though irrational and inappropriate, is a fact of life, and in some degree it is a part of all individual's lives. Consequently, every clinician must be aware of this dimension of his patient's problem. He should be able to recognize and understand anxiety, so that he can deal with it constructively.

COMMON ANXIETIES OF DENTAL PATIENTS

Anxiety and Pain

Pain serves a purpose. It is a warning of danger to the body so that the person can take protective action. Anxiety becomes the psychological substitute for pain. Through experience and associative processes, anxiety protects the organism by the anticipation of danger so that the organism can act before it is actually injured; it stimulates defensive and avoidance reactions. When the individual is forced into an unavoidable situation, such as going to a dentist, anxiety may run rampant, provoking tension and profound emotional changes even though the person has not been and will not be hurt. Anxiety greatly exaggerates actual painful experiences. It lowers the pain threshold and it increases the tolerance to medication. Pain, therefore, has its anxious and anticipatory aspects and these must be recognized and dealt with.

Anxiety and Body Damage

Concern about damage or mutilation of the body represents one of the child's most basic anxieties. Lack of experience and perspective makes trivial traumas, such as a slight cut or the sight of blood, seem catastrophic. Normally the adult learns to view his body more objectively and with greater emotional distance, and to have confidence in its toughness and resiliency. In the immature person, however, who still has a marked preoccupation with body integrity and body damage, just the thought of a needle, a scalpel, an injection, or a cut can create vivid imagination of body damage which can lead to anxiety severe enough to cause a major problem in management and treatment (Fig. 2–1).

Anxiety and Body Loss

Closely related to concern about body damage and mutilation is the concern about

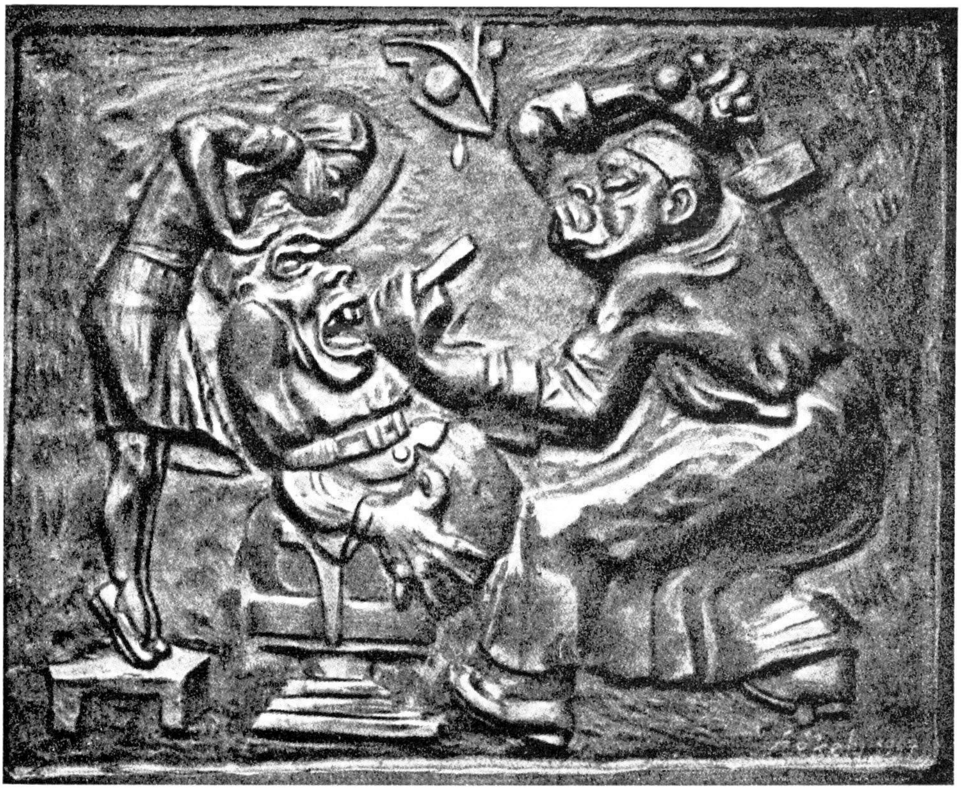

FIG. 2–1. The dentist as a surgeon. The Hungarian dentist, physician and artist IMRE SZEKELY 1898—) made this bronze relief in Budapest in 1947; it reflects a fearful patient's image of a dentist performing a surgical operation on the jaw. It is at first reminiscent of medieval art in its subject and style, with the dentist brutally hewing away in the mouth of a bound patient, but on closer examination we see that we are in a modern clinic, with a cylinder chair, an electric operation lamp, and a clinical assistant wearing a mask over her mouth. (Pindborg, J. J. and Marvitz, L., *The Dentist in Art*,* courtesy of Quadrangle Books, Inc.)

the completeness of the body image. Freud brought to our attention the child's concern about his body and its completeness when he described "castration anxiety" and "penis envy." However valid or common such feelings and fears might actually be, there is no question that the child is concerned about his body, its appearance, beauty, strength, and completeness.

This continued preoccupation with and desire for body perfection, beauty, and completeness is referred to as narcissism. Everyone has to some degree a narcissistic investment in his body; he wants to preserve it intact and keep it attractive. This aspect of life is obvious in wounded pride and self-esteem when a person grows bald, or loses his virility or athletic prowess. Likewise, loss of teeth and need for dentures may be of profound emotional significance. It can mean to a person that he is growing old, falling apart, or no longer quite complete.

Therefore, while removing teeth or constructing dentures may be a relatively simple technical problem, psychologically it may be far from simple. To the patient such changes may be quite unacceptable and unconsciously rejected, thus resulting in adverse reactions and complications.

Anxiety and Authority Figures

One of man's earliest and most basic anxieties is associated with parents who discipline and punish; the relatively small and helpless child has a dread of the relatively huge and powerful parent. This early perception of parent and associated anxiety is never completely outgrown. The early, archaic reaction pattern can be seen again when, for example, an individual is confronted by a powerful dignitary, such as a judge, or by a motorcycle policeman while speeding. The person experiences anxiety and acute discomfort unwarranted by the realities of the situation.

The dentist and physician too are symbolic of authority. They represent in the person's unconscious mind a familiar figure from the past who could hurt or damage. It is almost inevitable that a person entering a dentist's or physician's office will experience anxiety because of this unconscious association alone; symbolically he is walking into the room to face the powerful parent. The experience reactivates unconscious memories of that time when he, the child, was weak and the father (dentist) was powerful, when the father (dentist) could inflict pain but the child (patient) could not. Patients commonly unconsciously equate dental or medical care with punishment.

Therefore it is important for the dentist or physician to know that in his office, white frocked and with instrument in hand, he can and usually does arouse anxiety, solely on the basis of his symbolic significance as a figure of authority from the past.

Anxiety and the Sense of Helplessness

A major source of childhood anxiety is the inescapable fact that the child is small and weak in a world of powerful adults. This anxiety is overcome through such compensatory devices as independence and mastery. Mastery, independence, and control remain for most people important psychological defenses against the anxiety of helplessness and impotence.

Situations that tend to rob the person of his defense can create anxiety. A person surrenders a degree of mastery and control when he submits himself to the care of a professional person such as a dentist or a physician. This is enhanced when, for example, the patient lies down or sits in a semireclining position, when he is partially restrained, when his mouth is filled with sponges and a suction device, when he cannot talk or gesture, and when the dentist hovers over him with his "needle," "drill," or other instrument.

PERSONALITY TYPES

Personality is a structured pattern of behavior. The particular behavior pattern that a patient demonstrates suggests the personality type to which he belongs.

It is not necessary for a dentist to be a psychologist or a psychiatrist to identify a certain set of behavioral characteristics. However, it is necessary for him to be interested in his patient beyond his own area of special concern—the teeth and oral cavity. He must be aware of and make observations of the whole person, noting such things as the person's actions and manner, what he says and how he says it, his neatness and personal appearance.

There are several important and basic personality types that every clinician should recognize. The clinician should also understand the behavior and reactions of individuals belonging to each basic type: the oral, the compulsive, the hysterical, the paranoid, and the schizoid personality.

The Oral Personality

The person with this type of personality has more than the usual amount of emotional investment in the mouth and its function. The mouth and oral activity continue to be an important source of pleasure and a means of relieving tension. Consequently, eating, drinking, chewing, and biting are major preoccupations. Usually the person is obese, impatient, and tolerates frustrations poorly. He can be warm and friendly but his mood can quickly change, becoming biting, sarcastic, demanding, and unreasonable. The oral person is easily precipitated into a depression, and does not tolerate losses well. He is apt to experience much oral tension which may lead to unwarranted dental complaints or demands for dental attention which in reality are not essential. Recognizing the oral personality helps the dentist to recognize that some oral complaints are psychologically determined rather than representative of some actual oral pathology. Some patients with oral manifestations of psychological problems may need definitive psychiatric help, and a referral should be made.

The Hysterical Personality

The person with an hysterical personality tends to be emotionally labile, given to dramatic and histrionic behavior, suggestible and often highly imaginative. Seductiveness, coquettishness, and vanity are common features. Appearance is of dominant concern, and the person frequently appears overdressed. Such an individual frequently has severe anxieties and phobias, suffers from globus hystericus, gags easily, and tolerates manipulations in the mouth and throat quite poorly. However, the hysterical person is responsive to firm positive suggestion, and as a rule is rather easily hypnotized. Therefore, a kind, firm, soothing, reassuring manner may make the care and management of such a patient much easier than anticipated from the surface behavior of over-reaction and flightiness.

The Compulsive Personality

This type of person's dominant characteristics are perfectionism and rigidity. The individual is precise, punctual, meticulously groomed and concerned with details. The perfectionistic, inflexible characteristics make adjustments to change very difficult. The demands of such a person for repeated changes in the fixed or removable partial denture can drive a dentist to distraction. Even though the dentist fixes this, adjusts that, or equilibrates the occlusion, still the patient does not feel satisfied; something still seems out of line in the mouth. Unless the dentist is aware of the personality with which he is dealing, he can work endlessly to correct ostensible dental problems, when in reality the problems are in the personality. Not infrequently people of this type need psychiatric help.

The Paranoid Personality

The individual with a paranoid personality tends to be suspicious and distrustful. He presents himself in a guarded manner, and often raises questions about procedures which the average patient would accept without hesitation. The patient with a paranoid personality, lacking confidence and trust, is apt to be defensive and irritable, and on occasion displays unreasonable anger and blaming attitudes. Treatment of the patient with a paranoid personality should include caution; an attempt should be made to explain fully everything to be done, thus hopefully enlisting the patient's confidence and cooperation.

The Schizoid Personality

This type of personality is characterized by aloofness, a cold or distant manner. Frequently a pane of glass seems to exist between observer and patient, who tends to draw away and stiffen up with any possibility of intimacy or bodily contact. The schizoid person requires tact, patience and understanding, and the doctor must remember that the patient's behavior toward him is not personal but represents a deep insecurity in interpersonal relations.

SUGGESTIONS FOR THE PSYCHOTHERAPEUTIC MANAGEMENT OF DENTAL PATIENTS

The management of the anxious and emotionally upset patient may well constitute the dentist's major problem. Once he has gained the confidence and trust of the patient, carrying out the technical aspects of the dental care may be simple. Certainly the judicious and wise use of medication is a form of management of very great value. This technique of premedication, with clinical illustrations, is discussed in the following chapter. Here I would like to stress the value of relatively simple psychotherapeutic techniques which, with medication, can make dental treatment an easier experience for both the dentist and the patient.

Psychotherapy as used by the dentist will be largely supportive. The first steps in providing support are to anticipate anxiety and to be alert to its manifestations. A basic aspect of supportive therapy is the manner, the attitude, which the dentist presents. If he is warm, friendly, calm and unhurried, many perceptual distortions by the patient can be avoided.

The atmosphere of the office itself is also important. Attractive furniture, warm colors, a quiet atmosphere, pleasant background music, and friendly assistance can help put the patient at ease.

The dentist can be immeasurably helpful if he takes sufficient time to obtain the patient's confidence, approaching him with consideration, deliberation, and deft assurance. Explanations as to what he is going to do and what the patient may expect can be extremely helpful.

In supportive management of patients undergoing dental care, reassurance should be high on the list of the dentist's therapeutic techniques. Every person undergoing a crisis appreciates words of reassurance. Of course, they should not be inappropriate or misleading, but reassurance phrased in the context of appropriate explanations and clarifications can be most supportive.

Another therapeutic measure of great value is allowing the patient to talk about some of his feelings about procedures to be undertaken, about the loss of teeth, about the pain anticipated. Verbalization of feelings may bring relief, particularly when the person feels that what he is saying is fully understood and accepted without depreciation or ridicule.

A psychotherapeutic attitude is basically one of appropriate concern and respect for the total patient, an attitude which serves as a framework for all treatment. This attitude, plus technical dental skill, will assure the patient of good care and the dentist of the satisfaction of having cared for his patient in terms of his total needs.

Section II

Sedation, Local and General Anesthesia in Dentistry

Chapter 3
Sedation in Dentistry

INDICATIONS FOR AND PURPOSES OF SEDATION

People possess different capacities to withstand stress and, if the dentist cannot induce confidence in the patient and provide comfort by producing local anesthesia, then the local anesthetic must be supported with a drug that calms the central nervous system. However, we are definitely against the procedure of routinely administering a sedative or a narcotic to every patient who requires merely local anesthesia for a short, relatively simple operation. For lengthy procedures of restorative dentistry, the patient should be spared the simple stress imposed by the grinding and manipulation. Sedation is a "must" for any prolonged or severe oral surgery, such as multiple extractions involving any difficulty or the removal of impacted teeth with the patient under local anesthesia.

Let us now clarify the various purposes of sedation:

1. To allay apprehension, anxiety, or fear.
2. To raise the pain threshold.
3. To control secretion from salivary and mucous glands.
4. To control gagging.
5. To counteract the toxic effect of local anesthetics.
6. To control motor disturbances (as in cerebral palsy patients).[14]
7. To reduce tension and thus make it possible to obtain "centric registration" for patients who forcibly resist passive movements.
8. To reduce the stress associated with traumatic or prolonged sessions of surgery or restorative dentistry.
9. To stabilize the blood pressure for patients with hypertension or a history of cardiovascular or cerebrovascular disease.

THE "IDEAL" DRUG FOR SEDATION

Dentists treating ambulatory patients cannot follow the same procedures for the comfort of the patient as those used in the hospital. Hospital methods of premedication have, according to Dr. Wm. J. Mayo, "added so greatly to the comfort of the patient as almost to revolutionize surgical anesthesia."[10]

The ideal drug for sedation for the ambulatory patient, preliminary to administration of a local anesthetic, would depress only some of the specific higher centers of the central nervous system, bypass the medulla, and act and fade quickly without leaving a hangover, as do the drugs which we now employ. Such a drug is not available. However, a step toward the realization of such an ideal drug is seen in the development of neuroleptic-narcotic combinations even though these drugs are not yet adaptable for widespread use in general practice. Nitrous oxide-oxygen, considered as a sedative, is without doubt the safest, most nearly ideal drug available. The most reliable available statistics regarding its safety may come from Denmark, because there serious complications and deaths must be reported to the Department of Health. In 1970 1,500 analgesia machines were in use among 4,000 dentists, and since 1956 up to four million treatments had been administered under nitrous oxide analgesia without a single serious complication.

A short-acting barbiturate such as pentobarbital sodium, given in small doses, also comes close to serving the purpose. Pentobarbital sodium is a cortical depressant. In small therapeutic doses it acts as a sedative; in a larger dose it acts as a hypnotic.

THE CHOICE OF DRUGS FOR SEDATION

To make an intelligent choice of a drug which will safely produce specifically desired results, a basic knowledge of the pharmacology of the drug is absolutely necessary.

For this reason it is necessary for the dentist to possess a good knowledge of the basic anatomy and physiology of the central nervous system. A brief review, presented in general terms, follows.

The parts of the central nervous system affected by medication are the cerebrum, the thalamus, and the medulla oblongata.

The cortex of the cerebrum is the seat of consciousness, perception, and evaluation of incoming impulses which determine the active responses executed by the motor centers.

The thalamus is the substation for the incoming messages which are then relayed to the central cortex for further evaluation.

The medulla oblongata contains the nuclei for governing the unconscious vital functions such as respiration and blood circulation.

The main physiological characteristic of the brain is its requirement of a constant supply of oxygen. Even momentary interference of its oxygen supply, as, for instance, that caused by pressure on the carotid artery, will result in unconsciousness. Hypoxia will soon interfere with the medullary centers and anoxia lasting for a few minutes will result in irreversible damage to the central nervous system.

The drugs recommended for sedation and analgesia in the dental office are: (1) nitrous oxide and oxygen; (2) pentobarbital sodium; (3) meperidine, a narcotic analgesic; (4) scopolamine or atropine, both of which are members of the belladonna group, and (5) diazepam.

Nitrous Oxide-Oxygen

Among the methods which have been available to dentists is one with a long history, nitrous oxide and oxygen *sedation*. The real value of the use of nitrous oxide and oxygen as an "adjunct" to local anesthesia has been obscured by the claim that it should take the place of local anesthesia in restorative dentistry. However that may be, when nitrous oxide and oxygen are combined with the use of a local anesthetic, the gas provides for sedation and raising of the pain threshold. In many patients, including young children, the administration of nitrous oxide and oxygen will remove the fear and the sensation of the injections. A receptive patient experiences relaxation and a carefree, pleasant mood and some amnesia, while remaining conscious and fully cooperative. When the restorative procedure is over, the administration of pure oxygen for a few minutes will wash the nitrous oxide out of the patient's system. Shortly after the procedure the patient can leave the office unescorted.

The method cannot be used for patients who have an abnormal fear of losing consciousness. Neither is it successful for those who refuse to report their sensations to the dentist. Obviously it cannot be used for persons with nasal obstructions. However, if this method is not available or is not indicated, then the patient's fear and anxiety, or even at times phobia, can be allayed by other forms of sedation.

Nitrous oxide U.S.P. is a colorless gas with a sweet smell. It is available as a liquid in steel cylinders ranging from the easily transportable E cylinder to the large, heavy but more economical G cylinder. Nitrous oxide is relatively insoluble in blood and does not combine with hemoglobin, being carried in physical solution. It is largely excreted unchanged through the lungs with a small fraction escaping through the skin. Because the N_2O molecule does not dissociate in the body, its oxygen is not available for tissue respiration, but a glowing ember thrust into the gas will burst into flames.[8] Because of these properties, care must be taken to avoid placing any oil or grease on the reducing valves of the tanks. The gas when administered with 20 per cent oxygen is at best a very weak general anesthetic and when administered with at least 50 per cent oxygen will not depress the normal protective reflexes of the airway, or the vital centers of the medulla and the midbrain.

The term *sedation* is preferred to *analgesia* because sedation more accurately describes the achieved effects. To achieve true analgesia on a sensitive tooth, the patient must be brought very near the second stage of general anesthesia. Dentists should not bring patients into this stage unless they are trained and equipped to administer general anesthesia.

Pentobarbital Sodium U.S.P.

In small therapeutic doses pentobarbital sodium is a sedative, in larger doses a hypnotic, and further increments cause anesthesia. The barbiturates only slightly depress the protective reflexes until a large enough dose is given to produce respiratory depression.[8]

Meperidine Hydrochloride

Meperidine is an analgesic and not a very good hypnotic. It has some sedative value. Since it produces no immediately apparent subjective symptoms such as those occurring following the injection of a barbiturate, there is no definite warning indicating dose limitation.

The advantages of meperidine given with a barbiturate are: (1) Meperidine seems to have a synergistic effect on the barbiturate and has a sedative effect of its own. (2) Meperidine raises the pain threshold and gives the patient a sense of well-being, short of euphoria, even when administered in minute amounts.

The disadvantages of meperidine are: (1) It is a narcotic and its improper use can result in addiction. When it is to be used repeatedly in a specific case, the patient's appointments should be spaced a week apart; thus far no tolerance to the drug has been observed by us. (2) Meperidine should not be used for patients who are taking monoamine oxidase inhibitors (MAOI) such as isocarboxazid (Marplan), etc.[11] (3) It can act as a powerful respiratory depressant. (4) More dangerous still, it can cause serious cardiovascular depression. (5) Hypothyroid patients have an increased susceptibility to narcotics and may be poisoned by an otherwise safe dose of meperidine, since meperidine may be considered equigesic with morphine when given in a dose approximately 10 times that of morphine.[11] (6) Meperidine may cause a preliminary cortical motor stimulation resulting in some excitement, or it may stimulate the vomiting center producing retching and gagging. These latter effects are guarded against by always giving the barbiturate first.

Scopolamine Hydrobromide U.S.P. and Atropine Sulfate U.S.P.

Scopolamine and atropine have one common use in dental practice, to reduce salivary flow. According to pharmacologists such as

Innes and Nickerson, scopolamine acts as a respiratory stimulant to normal man under basal conditions but cannot be relied upon to counteract the effect of morphine-induced respiratory depression (p. 528),[8] while anesthesiologists such as Wollman and Dripps state that "the combination of scopolamine and a narcotic analgesia produce less respiratory depression than does the narcotic alone." They also find that "the combination of scopolamine with a barbiturate is subjectively more unpleasant than scopolamine plus a narcotic analgesic or atropine with a barbiturate or a narcotic analgesic" (p. 58).[8] Scopolamine is a good sedative and tranquilizer, particularly when combined with a narcotic analgesic. Its amnesic effect is dependable. The same dose, however, in case of idiosyncrasy may produce excitement ranging from restlessness through delirium. These effects are most often noted in the dental office in the very young or the aged. For patients in these age groups, the anticholinergic drug of choice is atropine.

Atropine, in the dosages used in intravenous sedation (0.3 mg normal adult) in dental practice, seldom produces any discernible effects except drying of the mouth. For the very young and the aged, the dosage is reduced. Reported effects of atropine in average clinical doses (0.4 to 0.6 mg) are a mild increase in the rate and occasionally the depth of breathing. Depth is probably increased through bronchiolar dilation and increased physiological dead space subsequent to mild vagal stimulation. A mild bradycardia (4 to 8 beats per minute) may result with no changes in blood pressure or cardiac output. Larger doses cause a tachycardia, most noticeably in healthy young adults, an age of highest vagal tone. Atropine and scopolamine have wide margins of safety but, because ordinarily therapeutic doses sometimes cause alarming reactions, the operator should be familiar with the symptoms and signs of idiosyncrasy. Finally, "Many semisynthetic congeners of the belladonna alkaloids . . . have been prepared. These have few advantages over the naturally occurring alkaloids and their derivatives and too many have already been marketed for clinical use."[8]

Diazepam N.F. and Other Nonbarbiturate Sedatives

Diazepam N.F. (Valium), promethazine hydrochloride U.S.P. (Phenergan) and hydroxyzine hydrochloride N.F. (Atarax) are included in the extremely long list of nonbarbiturate sedatives which have appeared on the market and been proposed as tranquilizers. "Their superiority over barbiturates is questionable." "It should be pointed out that nonbarbiturate hypnotic agents share most of the disadvantages of the barbiturates and have, in addition, the drawback that much less is known about their pharmacology and toxicology" (pp. 181, 121).[8]

Our clinical experience with promethazine and hydroxyzine combined with meperidine for intravenous sedation has only confirmed that in our hands they have no advantages over the barbiturates and are not as predictable.

Diazepam deserves further trial for clinical procedures which do not exceed 45 minutes. The best currently available source of information concerning the use of the drug in the everyday practice of dentistry is the SAAD Handbook,[13] which states that the principal effects of diazepam are: (1) muscular relaxation and reduction of muscle tone; (2) anticonvulsant action; (3) calming and tranquilizing effect and (4) amnesia. One should take precautions to see that the drug is: (1) not used for patients with glaucoma; (2) used with caution in elderly patients who may be confused; (3) not administered to those who must afterward drive an automobile or perform similar tasks while under its influence; (4) not combined with agents that produce additive or supra-additive effects such as alcohol, barbiturates, phenothiazines, MAO inhibitors and imipramine-like compounds.[8] One precaution must be reemphasized regarding the postoperative effect of diazepam. Although the drug provides an average duration of effective sedation of about 30 to 45 minutes, "it provides a pleasant postanesthetic euphoria; but this euphoria is more dangerous than that of the shorter thiobarbiturates. It may extend 6 to 8 hours after a 10-mg dose. The effect is not so much feeling capable of doing normal actions better, but of sheer irresponsibility."[13]

The use of tranquilizers has been adopted hopefully, but experience has shown that when these drugs are administered alone the results are unsatisfactory. These agents, used in combination with other drugs such as barbiturates and/or narcotics, may produce sudden unexpected depression of the respiratory center or an abrupt fall in blood pressure. We still prefer for sedation the use of nitrous oxide-oxygen, or barbiturates supplemented, when needed, with an analgesic, *e.g.*, meperidine with scopolamine.

METHODS OF ADMINISTERING SEDATION

Oral Administration

The simplest and safest route of drug administration is generally considered to be the oral one. In some instances it may be satisfactory; generally speaking, however, it has one severe drawback. Even for the same patient at different times, the effects are unpredictable both as to latency and optimum degree since they depend very much on the contents of the digestive tract.

If sedation is needed, a barbiturate such as pentobarbital or secobarbital, given orally 15 to 20 minutes before operation, will suffice in most cases. The dosage is determined by considering the patient's age, weight, and temperament. If the patient's tolerance to a drug is not known, it is wise to administer only half the average hypnotic dose, determined according to the age, weight, and temperament of the particular patient. If necessary, the dose is repeated after 30 minutes, and this regimen continued until the desired degree of sedation is obtained. For individuals with extreme apprehension, it may be well to reduce the amount of barbiturate and add meperidine or another narcotic in equivalent dosage. Depressant drugs should never be administered to the point that the patient passes the stage of deep sedation, that is, the patient must not be forced into hypnosis for he then is under general anesthesia with its attendant hazards.

According to Goodman and Gilman, the use of a barbiturate produces respiratory depression proportional to the dose of the barbiturate. At about three times the conventional hypnotic dose, the hypoxic drive is measurably affected by barbiturates while "the sensitivity of the medullary centers to CO_2 is affected little more than it is in natural sleep. However, the hypoxic drive persists at levels of intoxication causing complete insensitivity of the respiratory centers to CO_2" (p. 105).[8] In practice, one of us (N. B. J.) has seen two patients, both women about 30 years of age, go into coma 15 minutes following the oral administration of 100 mg of pentobarbital sodium. Thus is illustrated the great individual variation in response. The generally established rules of dosage, such as Clark's rule, Young's rule, etc., are not reliable for practical clinical use. A high-strung child of 6 or 7 years will not respond to a dose established according to weight or age. A person of advanced age may go to sleep after receiving 35 mg of pentobarbital sodium.

Intramuscular Administration

The intramuscular route is a more reliable one than the oral. The latency is fairly standard, but the individual's reaction to a "standard" dose is unpredictable.

Intravenous Administration

In our experience neither the oral nor the intramuscular route has proven as effective as intravenous sedation of patients. The manner in which the precise dosage may be titrated for each individual receiving the drug is the advantage of the intravenous route. By injecting the drug *very slowly* the dentist can obtain almost immediately an index of the patient's individual reaction to it, and the desired degree of sedation can be established.[1] Although the intravenous route is generally considered to be the most dangerous of all, if employed with optimum care it possibly is one of the safest.

Our experience with the intravenous route for the administration of pentobarbital sodium and meperidine with scopolamine *for sedation* to patients requiring extractions started in 1945 at the School of Medicine of Loma Linda University. The close cooperation of Dr. Forrest Leffingwell, Chief of Staff and Professor of Anesthesiology, and his guidance and suggestions have been of immeasurable help in this work.[9] Our introduction to diazepam first came through correspondence (1966) with D.M.G. Main, the Dental School University of Dundee, Scotland, followed later by personal visits with Main and his colleague J.I.M. Lawson. It was in 1966 that we first administered diazepam.

It should be pointed out that, in 1932, a dentist in general practice, S. L. Drummond-Jackson of London, was a pioneer in employing the intravenous route for administration of an *anesthetic* in general practice dentistry. Dr. Drummond-Jackson in 1962 reported that he had used the intravenous method of anesthetic administration for restorative dentistry and minor oral surgery for more than 40,000 operations without a fatality, nor had he had an emergency requiring the use of a resuscitant drug.[3,4] In 1934 Victor Goldman[7] published in a British dental journal the first English-language article dealing with the subject of intravenous anesthesia for dental surgery.

Inhalation Administration

Nitrous oxide-oxygen as a sedative or analgesic has been used again and again since 1868, when the two gases were first combined by Andrews, although he used them for anesthesia. Our interest in nitrous oxide-oxygen sedation was renewed in 1956 when one of us (N. B. J.) lectured at the Royal Dental College in Denmark, his native land. One of the guests at the lecture was Henning Ruben, D.D.S., M.D., chairman of the Anesthesia Department at the Finsen Institute and Hospital in Copenhagen. Dr. Ruben's concern for the control of anxiety, fear and pain in dental practice was expressed through his willingness to train dentists in the use of nitrous oxide and oxygen analgesia at the facilities of the Royal Dental College, Copenhagen.[12] The course was required by law if dentists wished to use nitrous oxide-oxygen sedation in their practice. The machine employed was a modification of the Foregger and the German Dräger analgesia machines. It had continuous flow, was extremely accurate and had built-in failsafes. The failsafes were designed so that the machine delivered no less than $2\frac{1}{2}$ liters of oxygen per minute in combination with the desired amount of nitrous oxide, and shut off the nitrous oxide flow if the oxygen pressure became so low that $2\frac{1}{2}$ liters/minute of oxygen could not be delivered. A machine was purchased and transported for use in private dental practice and in teaching at Loma Linda University School of Dentistry. The combination of local anesthesia and nitrous oxide sedation was so effective that there was soon a demand for additional machines. At our (N. B. J.) request, the McKesson Company installed both failsafe and oxygen flush valves on the McKesson Analor, and these machines were used for teaching of dental students. We have required that all machines used in our practice, for teaching and demonstration, have these features. A recently available addition to the machines of several manufacturers is a whistle which sounds when the oxygen drops below a minimum flow of approximately $2\frac{1}{2}$ liters/minute.

As discussed in Chapter 7, the ideal time and place to learn the use of nitrous oxide-oxygen sedation is in the undergraduate curriculum, as soon as the students have the necessary foundation in the basic health sciences, particularly in the physiology of respiration. Students should use inhalation sedation skillfully and in the same matter-of-fact manner they use local anesthesia.

PROCEDURE

All patients should be in the supine or semisupine position when receiving any injection, local or intravenous. Bourne's[2] studies are relevant to these procedures. The same rule is followed when inhalation sedation is used. We have never observed fainting when the patient is under sedation, even in the semisupine position.

Nitrous Oxide and Oxygen

When administering nitrous oxide-oxygen sedation, if the dentist is to know roughly the percentage amounts of inhaled gases, the air vent on the nosepiece must be closed. To assure adequate ventilation, the bag is first filled with oxygen and the oxygen flowmeter set at 10 liters/minute, a flow rate suggested by Drs. Gerald Allen and Gaither Everett of the University of Washington. The nosepiece is adjusted on the patient with the exhaling valve set to the least resistance.

After breathing oxygen for two minutes, the flow of nitrous oxide is set at one liter/minute and the oxygen reduced by one liter/minute. Thereafter, nitrous oxide is increased one-half liter/minute and the oxygen reduced one-half liter/minute keeping the total gas minute volume constant, until "base line" is reached. At base line, the patient reports a pleasantly relaxed feeling, and perhaps tingling in the hands and lips. Both before and during administration of the gases, the patient is asked to report the beginning of pleasant relaxation (base line). Furthermore, the patient is informed that by requesting more or less of the nitrous oxide, or by breathing through the mouth, he can always be in control of the level of sedation.

The first time a patient receives the gas, great care should be taken to proceed slowly. Rapid administration will frighten many patients because initial high concentrations of N_2O produce unpleasant rather than sedative effects.

The percentage of nitrous oxide needed to establish the base line for sedation varies between 10 to 40 per cent of the total flow of the two gases. At a constant total combined gas flow rate of 10 liters/minute the percentage of either gas is easily calculated. In our experience, as with that of Dr. Ruben,[12] the amount of nitrous oxide should never exceed 50 per cent; nausea, retching, and excitement are thus avoided.

After base line has been reached, such operations as scaling and curettage may often be accomplished without any complaint from the patient. Beyond this, the patient may experience pain. For this reason, local anesthetics should be routinely administered for those procedures which usually are painful, such as compound cavity preparations and any type of surgery. This is in keeping with the observation that nitrous oxide and oxygen in concentrations which bring about periosteal analgesia (which increases with concentration) produce little effect on tooth sensitivity, as tested by the Burton Vitalometer.[5]

There seems to be no limit, within practical consideration, to the length of time that patients may be sedated. It has been reported that "physiologic changes attendant to nitrous oxide-oxygen administration are closely related to administration of oxygen alone."[5]

There are few contraindications for the use of this form of inhalation sedation, even for so-called "risk" patients. The reason is that nitrous oxide is nontoxic and more oxygen is being administered with it than is inhaled in atmospheric air. It should not be administered to patients with nasal obstructions, acute infections or marked emphysema.

Summary

1. Start with the breathing bag full of oxygen and a flow of 10 liters/minute of oxygen.
2. Apply the nosepiece with the air vents closed and the exhaling valve open or freely movable.
3. Administer oxygen for two minutes, then add one liter/minute of N_2O and decrease the oxygen flow by one liter/minute. Thereafter, increase N_2O by one-half liter/minute increments and decrease O_2 by a similar amount, maintaining the previously established 10-liter respiratory minute volume of gases. Continue these adjustments until base line is reached.
4. When base line sedation is obtained, maintain the established flow of gases.

Pentobarbital Sodium and Meperidine

The technique for intravenous sedation, which follows, was taught to the first (1955) and each successive class of junior dental students at Loma Linda University, and has proved to be effective and safe. The students administer it whenever indicated (see page 21).

Pentobarbital sodium (Nembutal) is given first; a few drops are injected, followed by a minute's pause to watch for the appearance of any unusual sensitivity to the drug. The injection is continued at the rate of 10 mg every 30 seconds, while engaging the patient in casual conversation and keeping him under steady surveillance, checking the pulse and respiration, and observing the tension of the arm. The injection is discontinued when the patient seems relaxed and at ease. The patient should be brought into a state of light sedation. If this state does not seem sufficient to secure full comfort for restorative or surgical procedures, no additional barbiturate is injected because further injection could bring the patient into deep sedation or into hypnosis, beyond which stage general anesthesia could result. Instead, the lumen of the needle is aspirated to remove any trace of the barbiturate, leaving the needle in the vein. The syringe is then detached from the needle. It is replaced by a fresh syringe containing 25 mg of meperidine and 0.32 mg of scopolamine (see Fig. 3–1), which have been diluted with distilled water up to 5 ml to facilitate slow injection for the purpose of determining the exact point of sedation. During the injection the patient's pulse is checked and on the least indication of depression the injection is stopped.

Explanation of the Establishment of Light Sedation: "The Base Line"

One hundred mg (2 ml) of pentobarbital sodium are drawn into a 2-ml syringe. This is injected *slowly* as previously described, while maintaining verbal contact with the patient. The patient is carefully listened to and looked at to detect evidence of the first cortical symptom due to the action of the drug. The first sign may be a slight drowsiness or dizziness or a slight blurring of the vision. This stage is hereafter referred to as the "base line." The amount of drug necessary to establish this base line usually varies from 30 to 300 mg. After the base line is reached a variable amount of the pentobarbi-

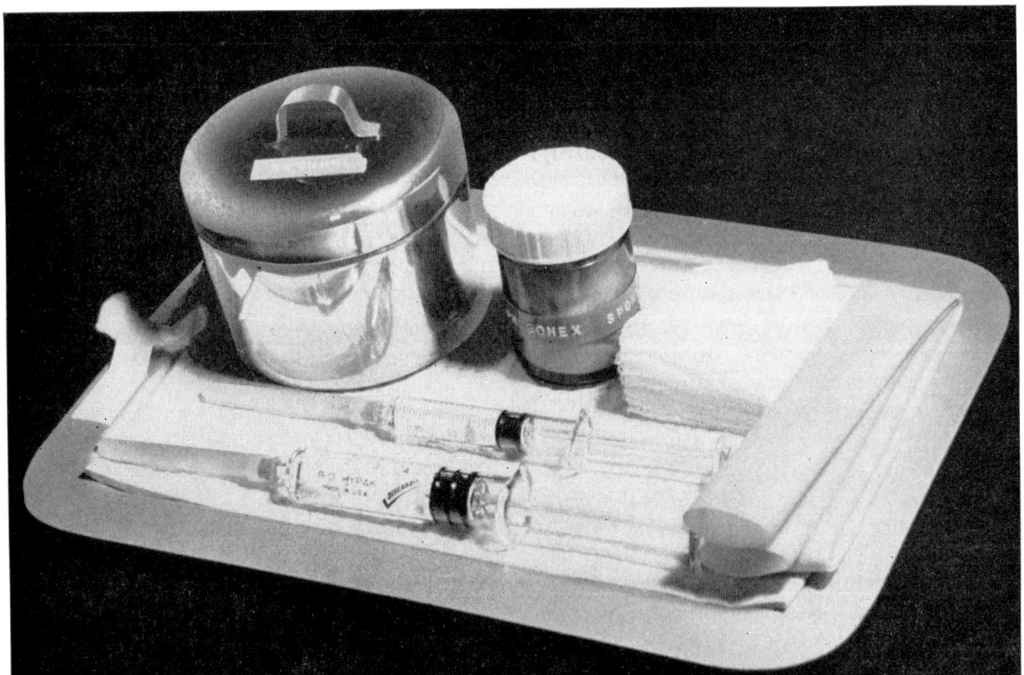

FIG. 3–1. Tray set up for intravenous premedication.

tal is injected, about 10 per cent. For instance, patients for whom this stage is obtained with from 30 to 50 mg are given from 3 to 5 mg more. But for patients who require 200 to 300 mg up to 20 to 30 mg more are injected. The amount of meperidine injected after this varies according to the amount of pentobarbital given: a patient who required 100 mg or more of the pentobarbital is given 25 mg of meperidine. If less than 100 mg of pentobarbital is given, then correspondingly less of the meperidine is injected; for instance, if 50 mg of pentobarbital has been used, then 12.5 mg of meperidine is given. In no case is more than 25 mg of meperidine injected. The technique is safe if followed with care and used as indicated (page 21). There is a total lack of tooth analgesia and only a mild degree of periosteal analgesia following such sedation, and therefore a local anesthetic must be administered to control pain.[6]

Summary

1. Inject the barbiturate slowly and watch the symptoms, especially the first time it is administered to a particular patient. Do not go beyond light sedation, which may require as little as 30 mg of pentobarbital sodium or as much as 300 mg. A once-established satisfactory and well-tolerated dose of a barbiturate given intravenously remains relatively constant for several years for the same patient.
2. If giving meperidine, use from 5 to 25 mg only. Dilute the 0.5-ml, 25 mg quantity of meperidine with sterile water up to 5 ml, then inject slowly.
3. Have oxygen and the necessary equipment for its administration ready for instant resuscitation, and know how to use the equipment.
4. Have at hand a pressor drug—phenylephrine (Neo-Synephrine), mephentermine, or a similar preparation—to treat a serious drop in blood pressure.

Diazepam

The first consideration in administering diazepam is that the patient be healthy with readily accessible and large veins. The patient must be supine. It is customary to inject 2.5 mg every 30 seconds until ptosis, which is equated with adequate sedation, is observed. Not more than 20 mg is given at any one setting. In patients for whom diazepam sedation is not sufficient in the recommended dosage, the barbiturate technique previously described is a useful alternative.

As with the intravenous injection of barbiturates, there is no standard dose which will produce the optimum sedation in each individual.

The dentist who wishes to administer diazepam should consult the excellent description of its clinical use in the SAAD Handbook.[13]

VENIPUNCTURE

The technique of venipuncture, in general, is not difficult to master. The median cephalic vein (Fig. 3–2*A*), veins in the forearm or on the dorsum of the hand should be chosen rather than the median basilic vein (median cubital). The median basilic vein, although often prominent and a tempting target for the novice, lies immediately over the brachial artery and median nerve (Fig. 3–2*B*). The artery has been accidentally injected into with results as severe as gangrene, requiring amputation. An extravascular injection of solution along the median nerve can cause long-lasting neuritis. Furthermore, there is a significant occurrence of aberrant superficially placed arteries in this area. On the flexor surface near the wrist, the ulnar and radial arteries are at risk, the latter particularly so, in the anatomical "snuff box." Even though there is a risk of hematoma when injecting on the dorsum of the hand, it should be considered a safe area for injection because the arterial network lies relatively deep. Most patients requiring intravenous sedation are so grateful for the relief sedation produces that they will overlook hematomas, if the possibility of a hematoma is carefully explained preopera-

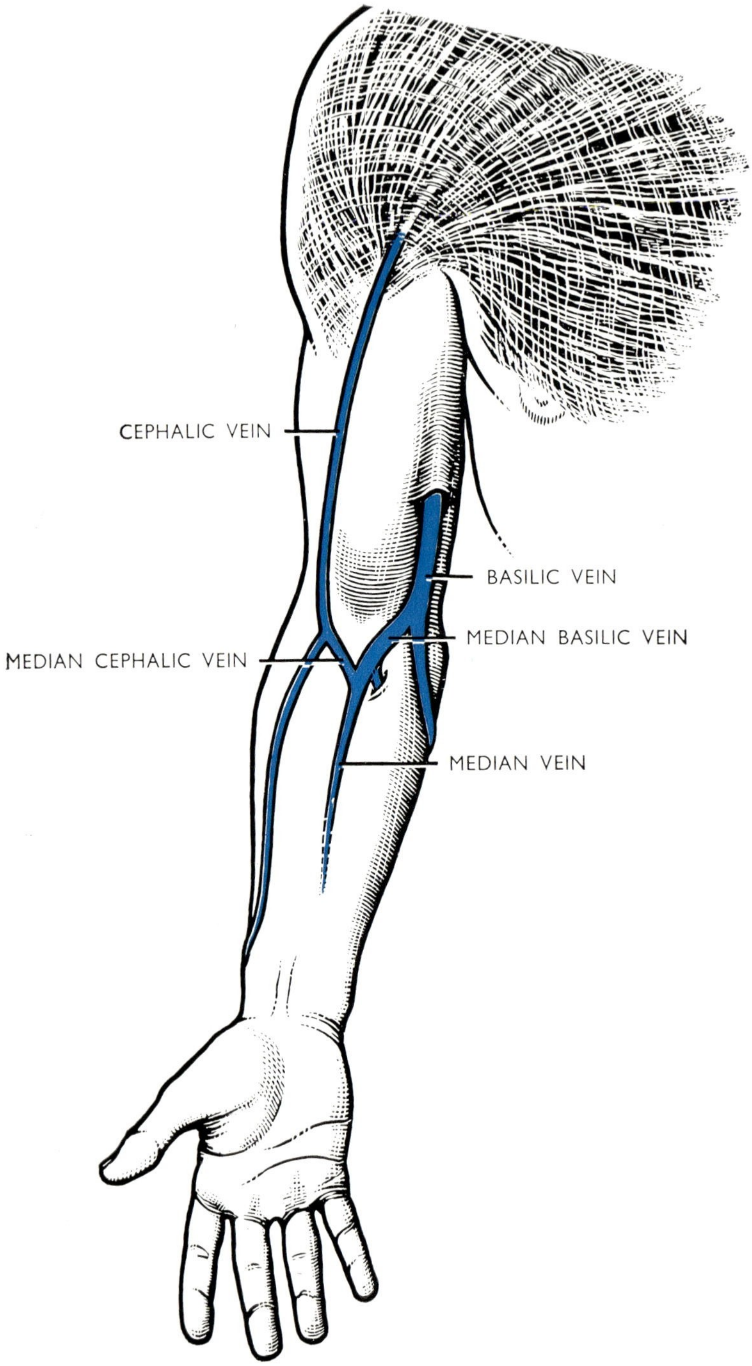

A

FIG. 3–2. See legend on opposite page.

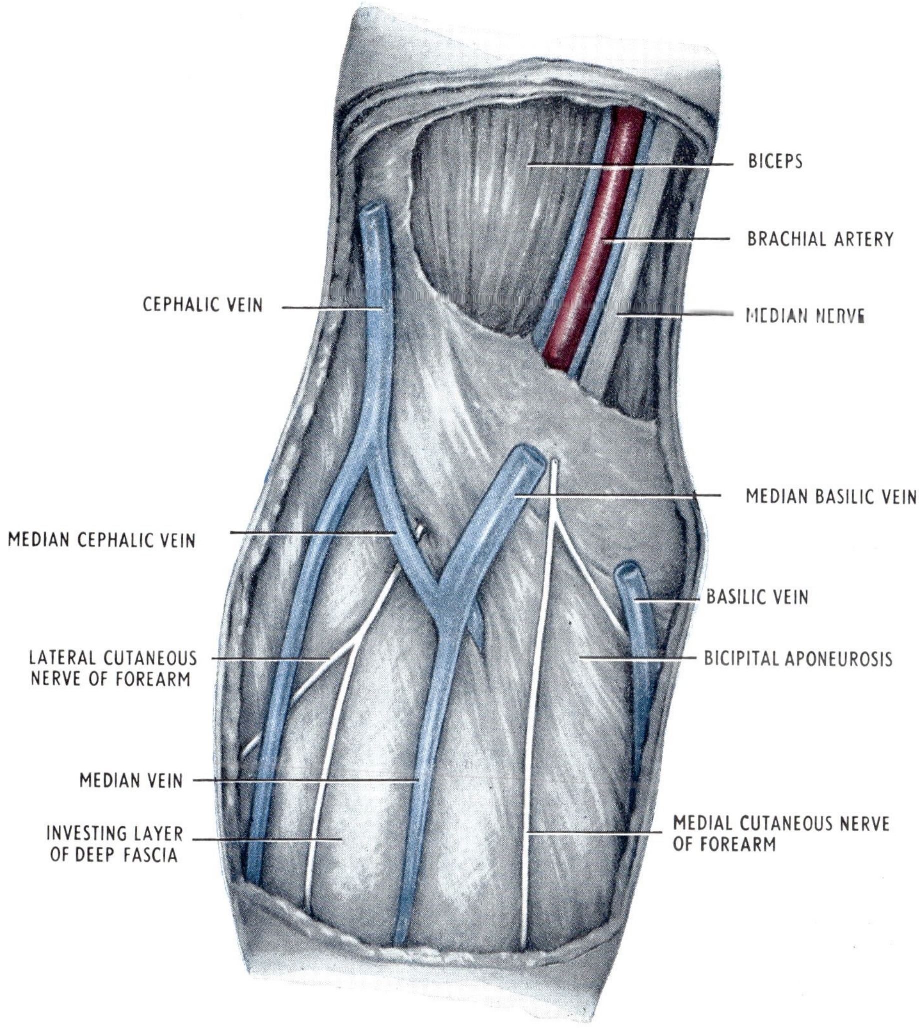

B

FIG. 3–2. *A:* The basic pattern of the subcutaneous veins. *B:* The brachial artery and median nerve lie deep to the median basilic vein. (Courtesy of Professor R. J. Last, Royal College of Surgeons, and Society for the Advancement of Anesthesia in Dentistry, London.)

tively. Disposable 25–21 gauge needles approximately 1″ to $1\frac{3}{8}$″ in length can be placed accurately in palpable superficial veins with a minimum of extravascular injections, hematomas or thrombophlebitis due to irritation of the intima. It is often difficult to keep the needle point from penetrating the lower wall of the vein with a conventional syringe and needle. To overcome this difficulty, one may employ a syringe with an offset hub, a D. J. winged adapter[13] or an Abbot Butterfly Infusion Set.*

The needle should enter only superficial veins. The skin is cleansed and a tourniquet is applied an inch or two above the puncture point. The tourniquet should be tight enough to stop the venous flow, but loose enough to allow some arterial circulation. In difficult cases a blood-pressure cuff maintained at 10 mm above diastolic pressure will gradually cause the venous return to fill the superficial veins. The patient clenches his fist to make the vein stand out; the operator stretches the skin distally which helps to immobilize the vein. Keeping the overlying skin stretched facilitates the puncturing. The skin is penetrated by the needle with the bevel up and away from the vein. The wall of the vein is hooked with the point of the needle, the wall is punctured, and the needle advanced a centimeter or more into the vein. Blood is aspirated into the syringe to determine that the needle is in the lumen of the vein. The tourniquet is then removed and the drug injected.

Injecting into an artery must be avoided because serious complications due to arteriospasm may result. If there is doubt concerning the location of the needle the syringe is detached from the needle and the tourniquet is loosened; blood will then spurt through the needle if the needle is in an artery. Furthermore, a barbiturate or other irritating drug injected into an artery will cause the patient to complain of pain in his hand and the skin will blanch.

A less serious complication occurs if the needle slips out of the vein and the drug is injected subcutaneously. Subcutaneous injection may be attended with considerable stinging pain. Injection of 2 to 3 ml of a 1 per cent procaine solution will counteract the irritant effects. However, if any considerable amount of the drug has been injected, it is not safe to administer an additional dose intravenously. The delayed effect of the first dose, taking place 20 to 60 minutes later, may result in too deep depression.

BIBLIOGRAPHY

1. *Accepted Dental Therapeutics*, 33rd ed. Chicago, American Dental Association, 1969/70.
2. Bourne, J. G.: *Studies in Anesthetics: Including Intravenous Dental Anesthesia.* London, Lloyd-Luke (Medical Books) Ltd., 1967, Chap. 4.
3. Drummond-Jackson, S. L.: A milestone in intravenous anesthesia. Corresp. Brit. Dent. J. *113*:404, 1962.
4. Drummond-Jackson, S. L.: Evipal anesthesia in dentistry. Dent. Cosmos. *77*:130, 1935.
5. Everett, G. B. and Allen, G. D.: Simultaneous evaluation of cardiorespiratory and analgesic effects of nitrous oxide-oxygen inhalation analgesia. J. Amer. Dent. Assoc. *83*:129, 1971.
6. Everett, G. B. and Allen, G. D.: Simultaneous evaluation of cardiorespiratory and analgesia effects of intravenous analgesia using pentobarbital, meperidine, and scopolamine in combination with local anesthesia J. Amer. Dent. Assoc. *83*:155, 1971.
7. Goldman, Victor: "Evipan" in Dentistry. Dent. Mag. Oral Top., *50*:1153, 1933.
8. Goodman, L. S. and Gilman, A.: *The Pharmacological Basis of Therapeutics*, 4th ed. New York, The Macmillan Co., 1970, Chaps. 6, 9, 10, 15, 25.
9. Jorgensen, N. B. and Leffingwell, Forrest: Premedication in dentistry. J. Southern Calif. Dent. Assoc., *21*:25, 1953.
10. Lundy, J. S.: *Clinical Anesthesia.* Philadelphia, W. B. Saunders Co., 1942, p. vii.
11. Modell, Walter, ed.: *Drugs of Choice*, 1970/71. St. Louis, C. V. Mosby Co., pp. 213, 205, 206.
12. Ruben, Henning: *Grundlag for Universal Analgesi.* København, Dansk Tandlaegeforening, 1958. (*Basis for Universal Analgesia.* Copenhagen, Danish Dental Society, 1958.)
13. SAAD: *Intravenous Anesthesia* (S. L. Drummond-Jackson, ed.), 4th ed. London, Society for the Advancement of Anesthesia in Dentistry, 1970.

* Abbott Laboratories, North Chicago, Illinois, 60064.

Films

14. Jorgensen, N. B. and Hurley, C. T.: Premedication for reconstructive dentistry of the adult cerebral palsy patient. 16 mm, sound, color, 20 min. Chicago, Amer. Dent. Assoc. Film Libr. 1957.

15. Jorgensen, N. B.: The comfort of the patient in dental practice. 16 mm, sound, color, 12 min. Chicago, Amer. Dent. Assoc. Film Libr. 1960.

Chapter 4

Infiltration and Nerve Block Techniques

THE ART OF LOCAL ANESTHESIA

Requirements of the Art

When we talk about the "healing arts" we consider both medicine and dentistry. The practice becomes an art if it is based upon (1) a disciplined approach to the knowledge of anatomy, physiology, and pharmacology, (2) the aptitude of the operator, and (3) the operator's dexterity in the use of his equipment and the materials of the particular field and a systematic application of his skill, and (4) the careful consideration of the requirements of the individual patient.

Upon these prerequisites rests the possibility of refining a mere craft into the higher level of an art. It takes discipline, assiduity, and a sacrifice of time and energy on the part of the practitioner. However, the time invested in such a disciplined approach is regained manifold when local anesthesia is obtained which results in the composure of the patient and a relief of the strain of the dentist's own nerves.

Anesthesia in Medicine and Dentistry

The medical profession has developed anesthesia into a great art during the last thirty years. Oral surgery, too, has made great strides in developing methods for pain control to a high level. Only the dentist in general practice seems to be marking time, for little progress in pain control has taken place during the sixty years since the synthesis of Novocain (procaine). We must remember the difference between the modern execution of anesthesia in surgery and anesthesia in dentistry. Medical anesthesia has become a distinct specialty, whereas in dentistry the dentist usually has been both operator and anesthetist. Furthermore, in general dentistry there has been a tendency to aim toward more and more simplified "techniques," often disregarding anatomical variations from an "ideal average," which in reality does not exist. Meanwhile all other branches of the healing arts have been striving for refinement and more exactness. The result is apparent: our methods of anesthesia are not regarded with favor by the general public. The available methods of controlling apprehension and pain are so little understood by dentists and the public that many people do not avail themselves of any dental health service and another large group will accept only dental extractions under general anesthesia.

Nobody likes needle pricks, and there may be more apprehension concerning needles entering the oral cavity than is aroused by injections in any other part of the body. Even if the injection is given painlessly, still the feeling of the solution being injected, and of the advancing of the needle, cause proprioceptive afferent impulses. These impulses lower the pain threshold and may lead to severe emotional disturbance.

Principles of Nerve Block Administration

Injections *can* be given without the transmission of sensory impulses. The anesthetist must know the relative sensory qualities of the different structures involved. The mucous membrane is pain sensitive; the loose, fatty areolar fill-in tissue possesses little pain sensation; tendons and muscles are pain sensitive. Accordingly the pain-sensitive structures should be avoided by the needle, or, in the case of a structure such as the periosteum, which must be touched, the site should be anesthetized before the needle reaches it. The awareness of the needle's progress can be avoided if it is advanced by steps. At each step, stop and inject a drop or so of the anesthetic solution, waiting five or six seconds before proceeding.

For nerve blocks use a needle heavy and rigid enough to be used as a probe, which as it is advanced by steps guides the anesthetist to the area next to the nerve without injuring the trunk; injections should always be given slowly to avoid tissue injury, and only a minimum optimum amount of the solution should be injected, thereby minimizing the chances of either local or systemic side effects.

The principles of diffusion govern the success or failure of local anesthesia. If a barrier is situated between the injected solution and the nerve trunk or nerves, then either total or relative failure may occur. Examples of such barriers are the interpterygoid fascia when giving the inferior alveolar injection, or the cortical bone and a varying thickness of the cancellous bone when giving the supraperiosteal injection. These barriers may be considered as semipermeable membranes. The amount of the solute (the dissolved substance) that will pass through this barrier within a fixed time depends upon the density of the semipermeable membrane and the concentration of the solute. The denser the membrane, the bone, or the fascia, the less of the solute will penetrate. The higher the concentration of the solute, the more will pass through. We can control, within practical limits, the concentration of the solute next to the barrier and the time element by injecting slowly.

Other important factors to consider in diffusion are the terms "cellular diffusion" and "turbular diffusion." Cellular diffusion takes place if the solute is left quiet, without being stirred; in this case the concentration is maintained at the place where diffusion is desired. If turbular diffusion occurs, the solute is disturbed by stirring as in a jar. For instance, if the injection is given rapidly or is followed by massaging over the area of the injection, the chance of a successful injection is evidently minimized. The solute will spread out into the solvent, the concentration will be lessened, and less of the solution will penetrate at a given point.

Preparation of the Patient

After a careful history is taken and before the local anesthetic is injected a few casual remarks are addressed to the patient, assuring him that the procedure will be painless. The chair is adjusted to place the patient in a semisupine position; the topography of the structures to be anesthetized is studied by palpation and observation. Now the area of injection is wiped with sterile gauze and a topical anesthetic is applied. After this has taken effect, the mucous membrane is again wiped with sterile gauze and the area is swabbed with an antiseptic.

Injections should never be given in an

unclean oral cavity. If necessary, prophylactic treatment should be given. If the area of needle insertion cannot be kept dry because of a copious flow of saliva, rolls of gauze are placed in the fornices of the buccal vestibules over the parotid duct and a pad of gauze is placed under the tongue to cover the submandibular duct.

EQUIPMENT AND MATERIALS

Progress in the field of local anesthetic administration, since the discovery of procaine, has largely centered about improved equipment and materials. The improvements for the most part have been made in the types of syringes and needles available and in the prepackaging of sterile needles and anesthetic solutions. These advances add immeasurably to the convenience and safety of the administration of local anesthetics.

Two types of syringes are used in dentistry. The first, the cartridge syringe, enjoys almost universal and exclusive acceptance. Its latest improvements consist in its sideloading capability and provision for aspiration. The second, the all-glass Luer-Lok syringe, is seldom used. Glass syringes have been almost entirely displaced by presterilized, disposable, plastic syringes with or without attached needles (Fig. 4–1).

Stainless steel needles presently available largely eliminate the danger of breakage. Two main types of needles are needed for dental injections: 23-gauge, $1\frac{5}{8}$-inch needles for deep injection and 25- to 27-gauge, 1-inch needles for supraperiosteal injections. Unfortunately, most manufacturers do not produce the 23-gauge, $1\frac{5}{8}$-inch needles owing to

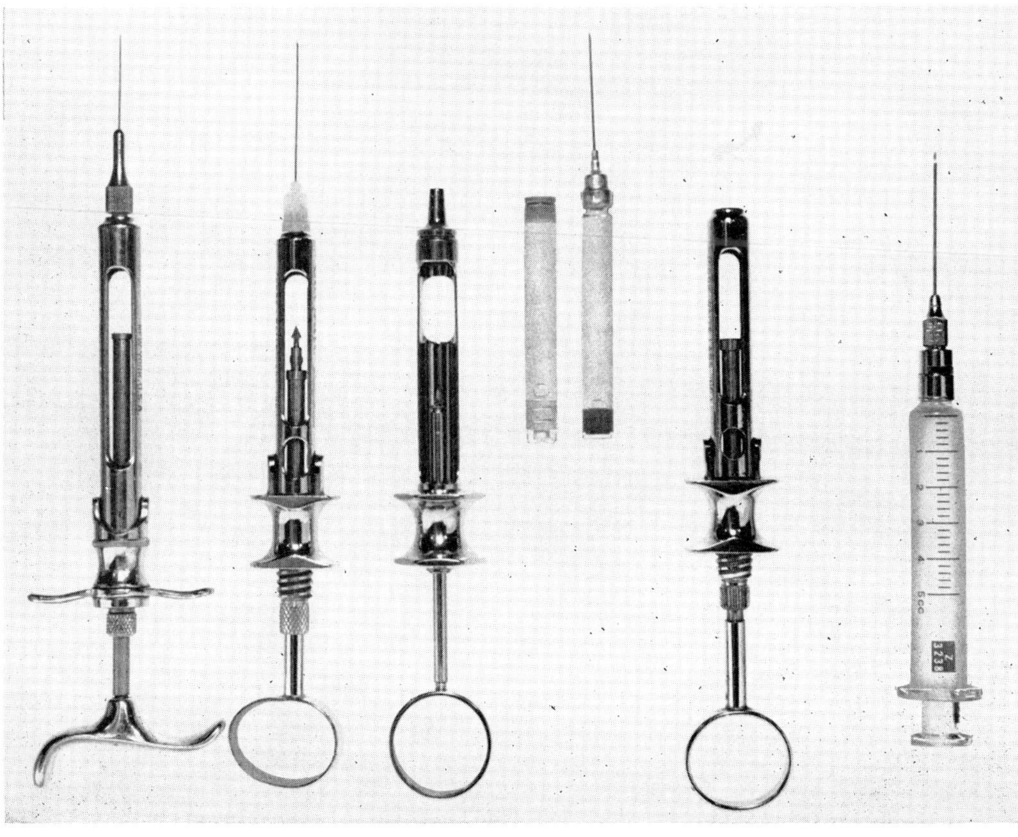

FIG. 4–1. Syringes in general use. (Courtesy of Cook-Waite Laboratories, Inc.)

the lack of demand for them. Dentists almost universally assume that the thinner the needle, the less discomfort there is to the patient. The truth is that any deep injection can be given painlessly with the heavy needle. Ample demonstration of this truth is given in the student dental clinics of Loma Linda University and in the teaching films produced at the University.[15–18]

Many authorities[3,4,9,10 11 13] state that a heavy, rigid needle is necessary to accomplish nerve block injections precisely, since the needle must be used as a probe (see page 71). Furthermore, the needle point must be sharp and short bevelled to glide easily along the periosteum and to avoid puncturing blood vessels (Fig. 4–2). The Mizzy Corporation and Cook-Waite Laboratories, Inc., have manufactured such needles (see page 86).

Sterilization of syringes and needles requires autoclaving or dry-heat sterilization. Autoclaving is done at 121° C (250° F), usually for 30 minutes. Dry-heat sterilization requires that an internal temperature of 160° to 180° C (320° to 355° F) be maintained for at least one hour. The higher temperature is preferred.[1] Only long, heavy needles can be safely sterilized for further use. Before sterilization, these needles must be cleansed with a stylet, flushed with a detergent or ether to remove all organic matter, and rinsed first with alcohol and then with water. Until presterilized disposable needles satisfactory for nerve block injections are available, these procedures for sterilization must be followed. Alternatively, after sterilization and one use the heavy, rigid, needles may be discarded.

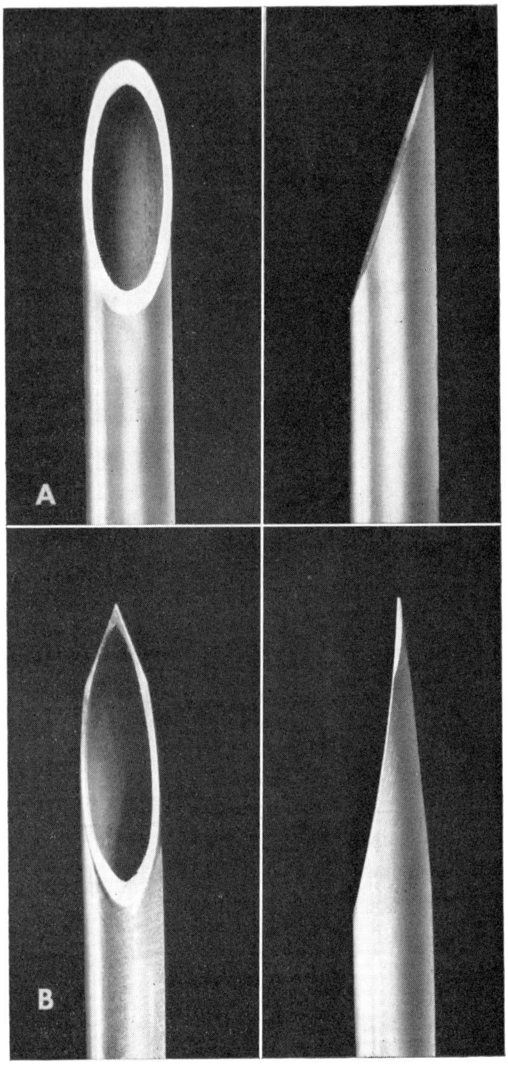

FIG. 4–2. Preferred sharp needle points: *A*, Short bevelled. *B*, Huber. (Courtesy of Cook-Waite Laboratories, Inc.)

DIMENSIONS AND STRUCTURES IMPORTANT TO ANESTHESIA OF THE MAXILLARY NERVE AND ITS TERMINALS

It is evident that knowledge of the dimensional variations is important whenever deep injections are intended, and this will be brought out in the discussions of the different nerve blocks. The technique of local anesthesia must be based upon a thorough knowledge of anatomy if it is to be considered and practiced as an art and a science. "Average" depths of insertions and directions of needles do not exist, as is evident by an elementary study of morphology. Glance at Figures 4–3, 4–5, and 4–7 and see the enormous variance in the sizes of the skulls and the great variance of thickness and density of the bone. The cancellous and cortical bony structures around the root apices determine the success or failure of the simplest of all injections, the supraperiosteal.

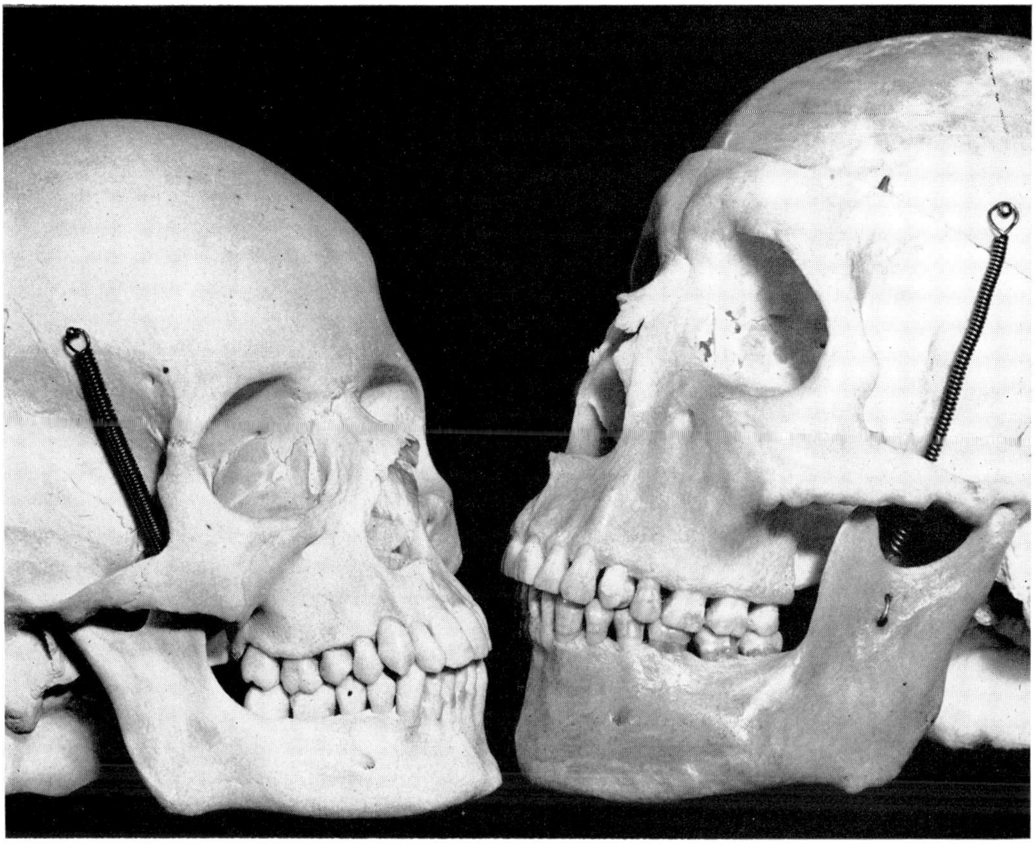

FIG. 4–3. The variation in size of unblemished skulls.

Figure 4–4 illustrates the maxilla. The roots are covered in some areas by paper-thin cortical bone and in other areas are completely bare. A supraperiosteal injection in the completely bare areas would without fail produce anesthesia by infiltration. But examine the other extreme, Figures 4–5 and 4–6. One skull is from an adult and one is from a 6- to 7-year-old child. In both subjects the root apices are covered by a 1-cm thickness of bone, and the cortical layer of bone is thick and dense. No amount of solution deposited against this bone would produce anesthesia of the dental plexus of nerves. An absolute diagnosis of these bony variations may be difficult to make. Whenever the root contours can be felt by palpation, a fairly thin bony covering of the roots may be predicted (Fig. 4–4), but the density or porosity of the cortical bone cannot be ascertained except by the trial-and-error method. The permanent first molar in the young child is covered by a layer of bone which is thicker than it will be in the adult state; with development the molar moves downward and forward, narrowing the distance between the palatine and outer bony plates. It may also be presumed that the root apices are closer to the outer cortical bone in a skull with a high maxilla than in one in which the maxilla is lower (compare Fig. 4–7*B*). Primary teeth are not easier to anesthetize than the permanent teeth. Notice in Figure 4–5 how smooth and dense the cortical bone appears to be. Also notice Figures 4–8 and 4–9 depicting the dissection of the maxillary and the infraorbital nerves and the alveolar plexuses. The latter lie high in the lateral wall of the antrum of this young skull because of the space occupied by the permanent tooth buds.

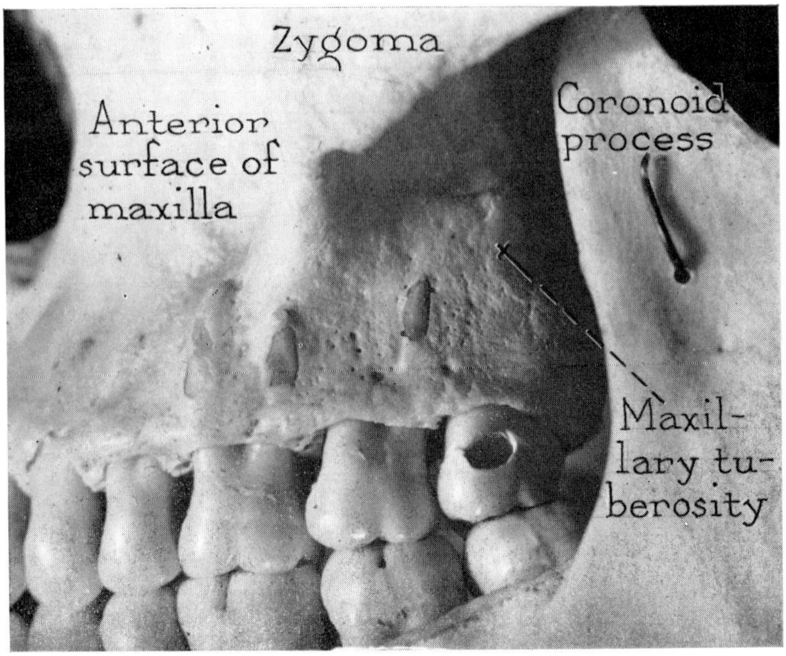

FIG. 4–4. The relation of maxillary permanent molar roots and cortical bone.

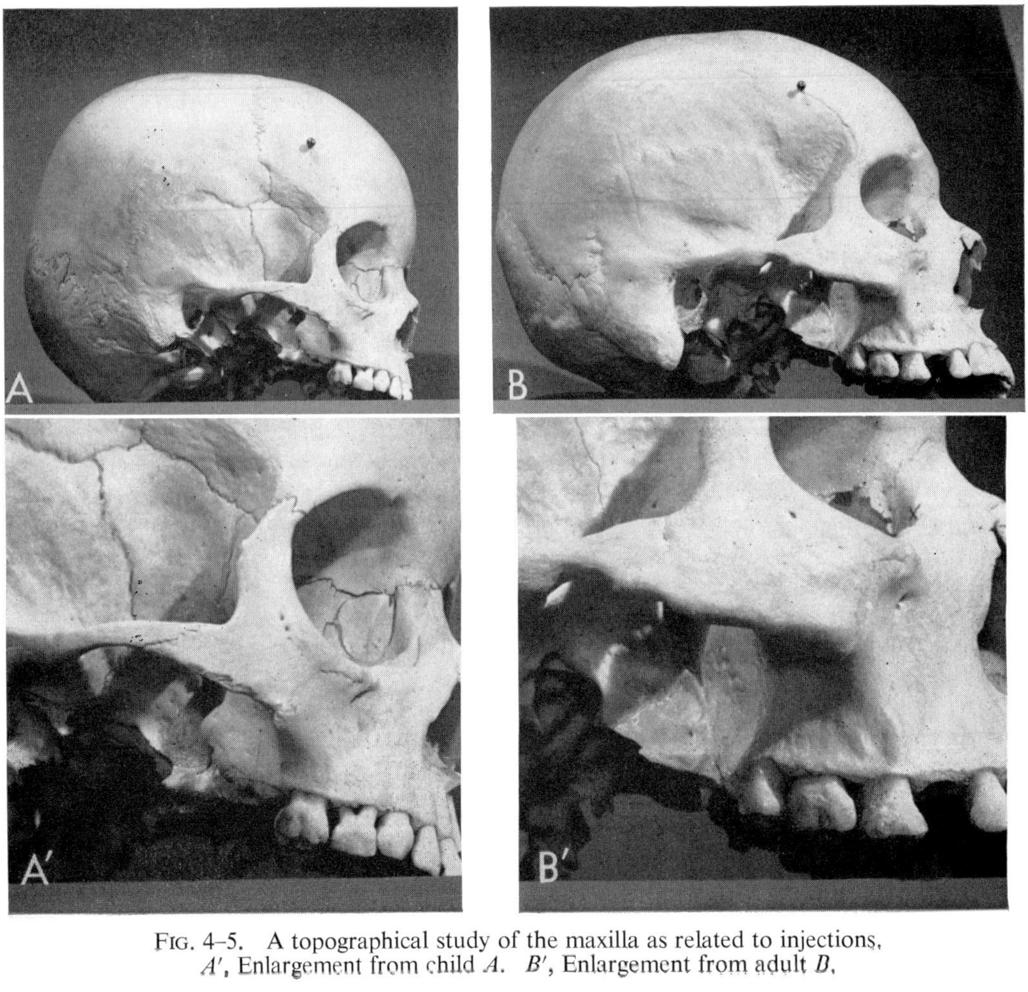

FIG. 4–5. A topographical study of the maxilla as related to injections. *A′*, Enlargement from child *A*. *B′*, Enlargement from adult *B*.

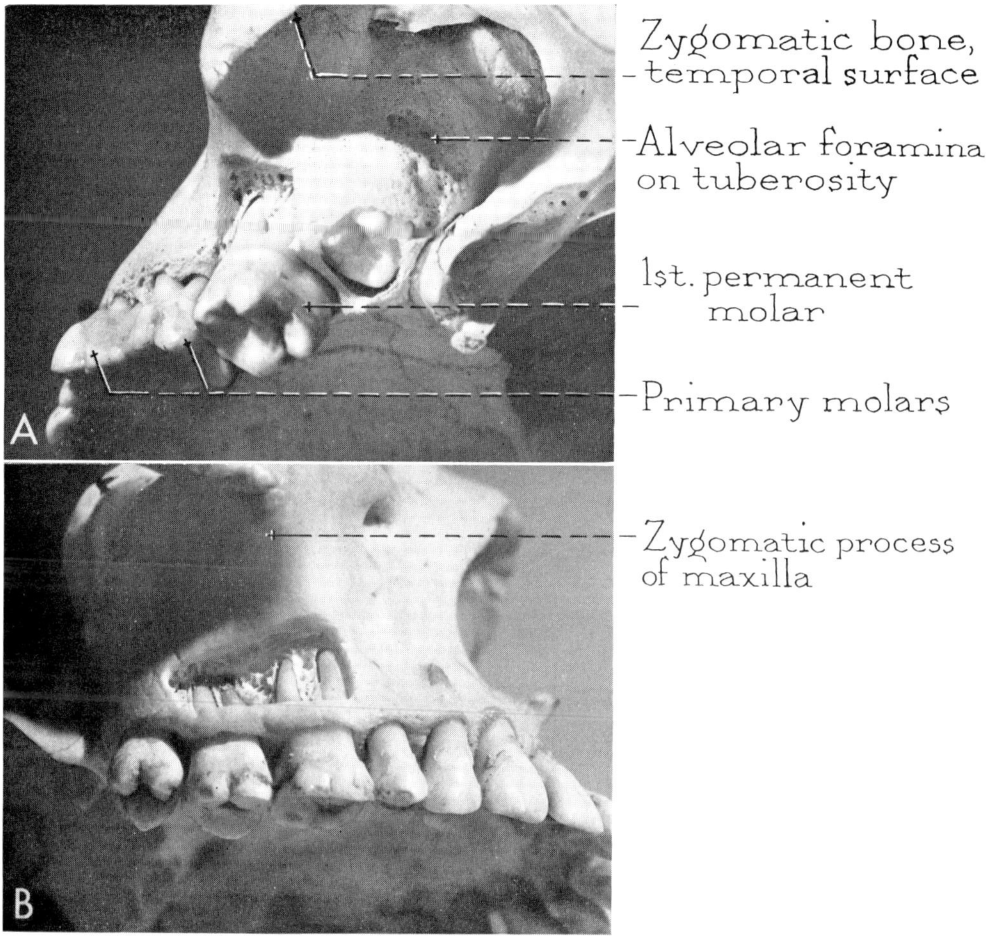

FIG. 4–6. Thick dense bone covering maxillary permanent molar roots. *A*, Child; posterior-inferior view. *B*, Adult; lateral inferior view.

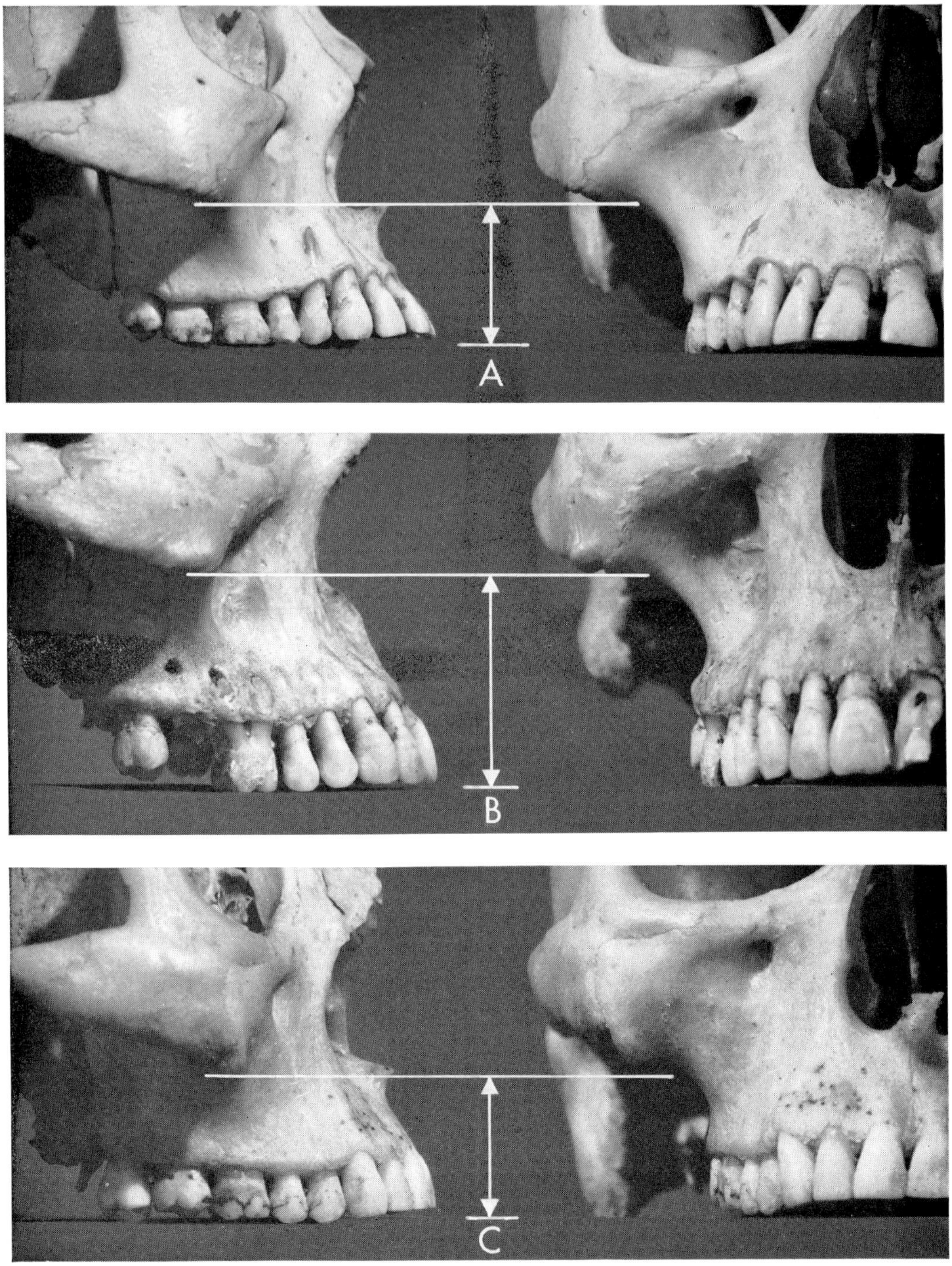

FIG. 4–7. A comparison of maxillary height and tooth-bone relations. *A*, Average maxilla. *B*, High maxilla. *C*, Low maxilla.

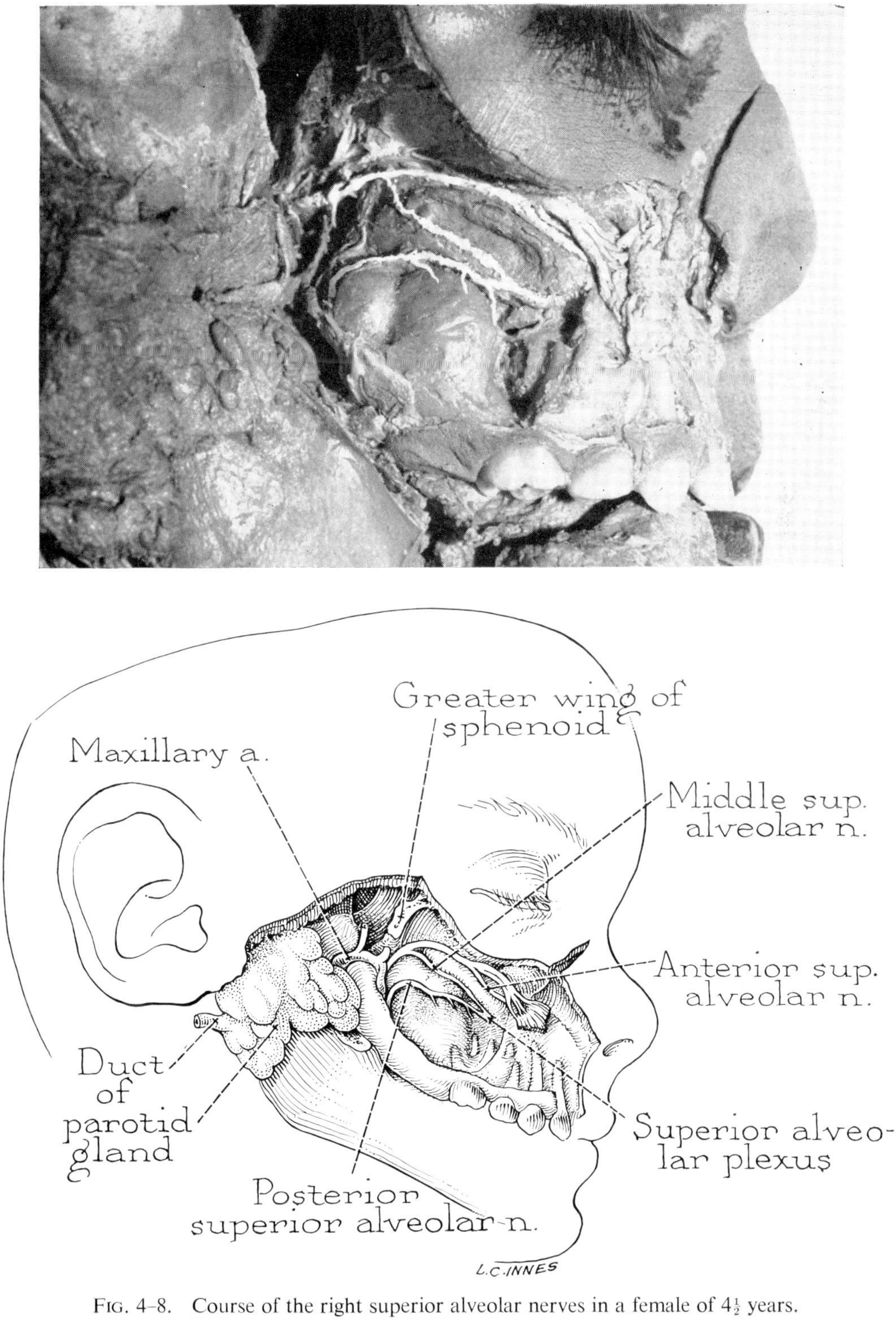

FIG. 4-8. Course of the right superior alveolar nerves in a female of $4\frac{1}{2}$ years.

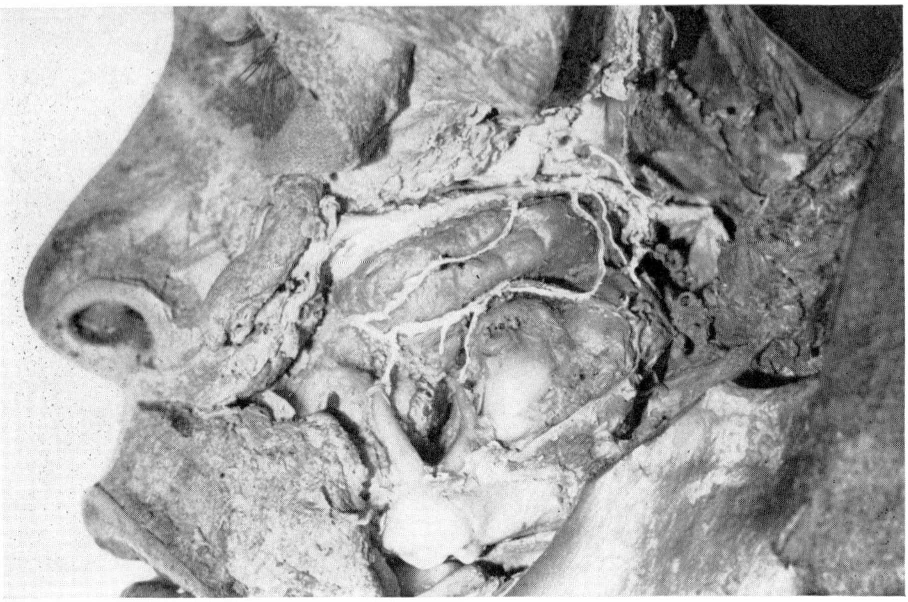

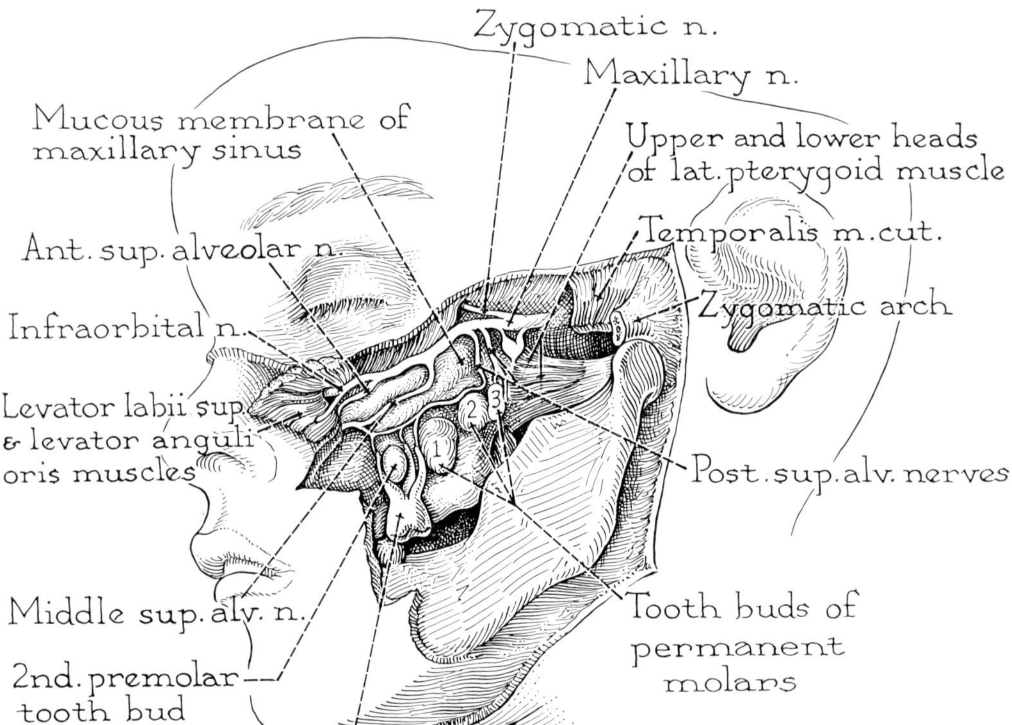

FIG. 4–9. Course of the left superior alveolar nerves in a female of 4½ years.

ANESTHESIA FOR MAXILLARY TISSUES

The Supraperiosteal Injection

Purpose

The supraperiosteal injection as described by Sicher[11] and by Fischer[4] is made to provide plexus anesthesia in favorable cases. When anesthesia of the pulp and hard tissues is intended, the term "infiltration anesthesia" is incorrect. Strictly, the method refers to the technique of injecting the solutions directly into the tissues to be treated. The terms "supra-" or "paraperiosteal" (Monheim[9]) or "plexus" anesthesia (Sicher[11]) are more appropriate. The terms mean that anesthetic solution deposited upon or along the periosteum must first diffuse through periosteum and cortical bone to reach the superior alveolar plexus of nerves lying in the cancellous bone. Generally the cortical bone covering the apices of the maxillary teeth is thin and perforated by many small openings; in other words it appears porous. According to the prior discussion of diffusion, the anesthetic solution will be readily carried to the dental plexus. Because it is the simplest of all methods used in dental local anesthesia, it is apt to be improperly given. The violation of the principles of physiology increases simultaneously the probability of partial or total failure and the possibility of unpleasant side effects.

Technique

Standard Approach. MORPHOLOGY. As you have observed in Figures 4–3 to 4–7 there is great variation in the smoothness, density, porosity and thickness of the cancellous and cortical bone surrounding the maxillary teeth. The apices of the primary teeth are covered by denser bone than those of the adult. The absurdity of making generalized statements in regard to the bone structure covering the maxillary teeth is well illustrated in Figure 4–6. The buccal root ends of a 6- to 7-year-old child are covered by bone almost 1 cm in thickness. Conversely, the root end of the adult's first premolar projects through the cortical bone, but the first and second molar root tips are covered by 1 cm of bone with a thick and dense cortical layer.

These illustrations of the maxilla demonstrate why the "infiltration" (a preferable

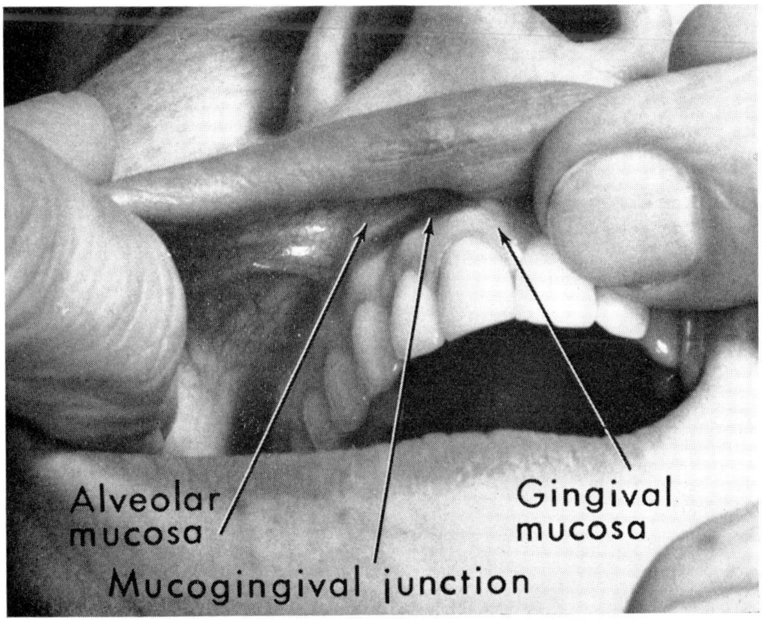

FIG. 4–10. The oral mucosa in a young adult.

term is "supraperiosteal") technique must fail at times. Failure requires that the anesthetist must be able to supplement the supraperiosteal injection with a nerve block.

PREPARATION OF THE PATIENT. The positioning of the patient and the preparation of the tissues for injection are described on page 36.

THE INJECTION. Hold the patient's lip and cheek between your thumb and first finger, and stretch the flesh outward so that the border line between the movable alveolar mucosa and the firm, fixed, gingival mucosa can be distinguished (Fig. 4–10). Make the needle puncture through the alveolar mucosa near the gingival mucosa; immediately deposit a drop of the local anesthetic solution here. Wait 4 or 5 seconds and then advance the needle toward the apical region of the tooth to be anesthetized. Inject a drop or two before contacting the exquisitely sensitive periosteum. To eliminate the danger of the needle sliding between periosteum and bone, direct the needle at an obtuse angle to the bone. The depth of insertion is only a few millimeters. The solution is deposited *very slowly* so that the tissue does not balloon. One-half milliliter of the solution deposited over two minutes of time gives the best result.

Modified Approach. When the supraperiosteal injection is ineffective owing to anatomical variations, a modified procedure will usually correct the failure. After preparing the tissue a small sterile cotton roll is placed in the fornix of the vestibule and held firmly against the mucosa with the first finger or thumb of the left hand. The needle is inserted and advanced by steps toward the periosteum (Fig. 4–11). The injection is given slowly, taking about 2 or 3 minutes to deposit no more than 0.25 to 0.5 ml. The tissue must not balloon. Use a solution containing a minimum amount of epinephrine to avoid after-pain or sloughing due to ischemia. The simple technique converts the alveolar soft tissue area into an almost closed space. The solution is directed to diffuse medially through the cortical bone instead of spreading into the facial soft structures. The marginal palatal gingiva, also, generally is anesthetized by this procedure.

Cautions

Theoretically, according to the discussion of diffusion (p. 36), the method can be used in all cases. But, because of the time re-

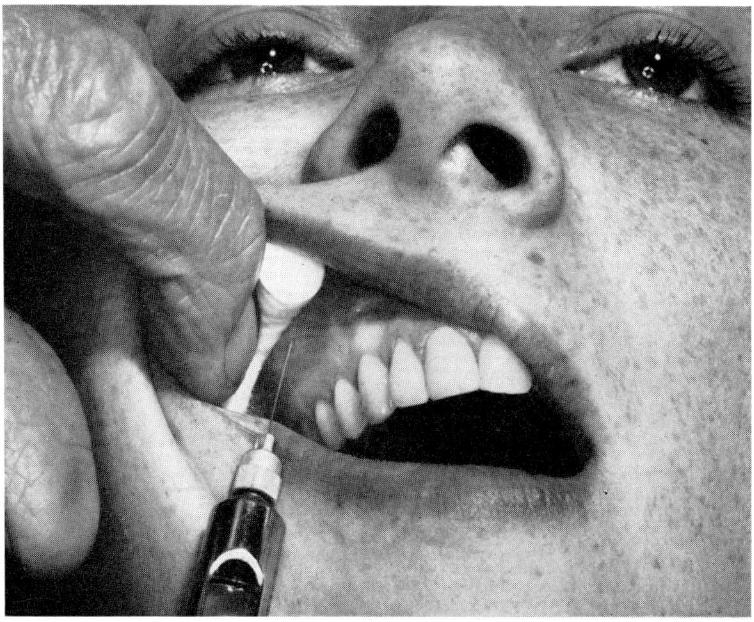

FIG. 4–11. The modified supraperiosteal injection.

quired, there is a point beyond which it is not practical or acceptable for the dentist or the patient. And, of course, this method should never be used in case of infection or acute inflammation.

Always practice aspiration and inject slowly in minimal volumes.

Finally, there must be further investigation to determine the effect of the concentration of the anesthetic solution and the vasoconstrictor on the tissue cells they bathe.

The Greater Palatine and Nasopalatine Nerve Blocks

Purpose

Whenever operations or trauma involve the soft structures palatal to the upper teeth, the greater palatine or the nasopalatine nerves or both must be blocked, depending upon the extent of the operation or surgical procedures.

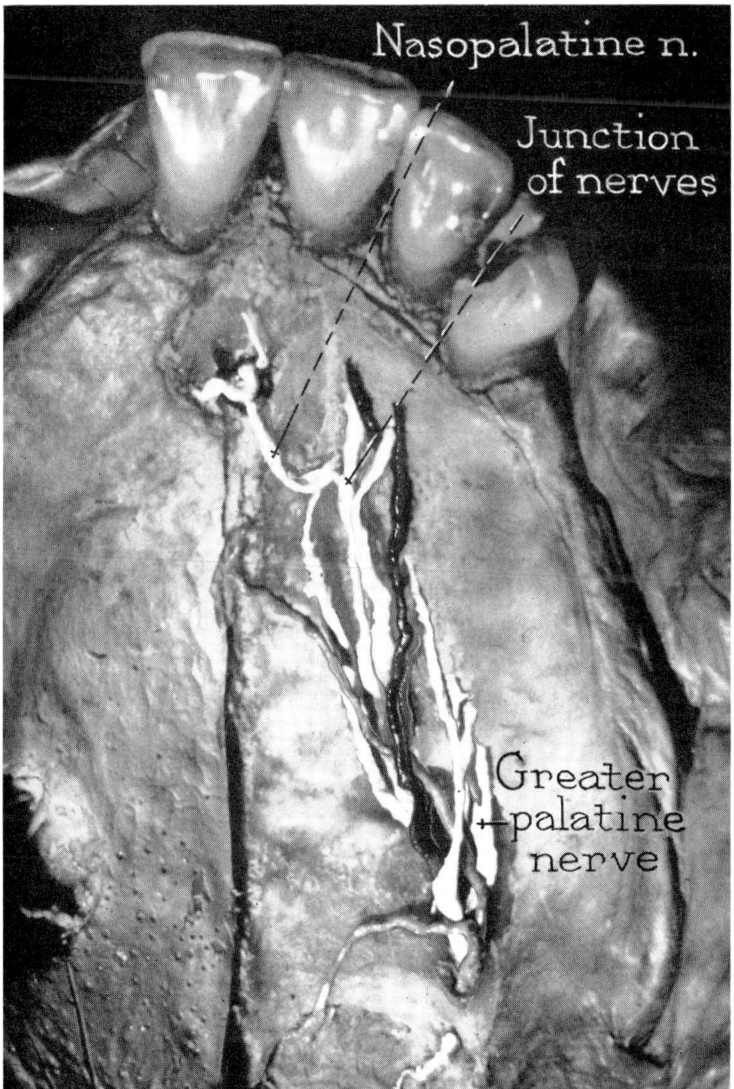

FIG. 4–12. The palatal course and the junction of the greater palatine and nasopalatine nerves.

Technique

Greater Palatine Nerves. MORPHOLOGY. The course of these nerves and their innervation are discussed on page 125. In Figure 4–12, observe the respective course of the two nerves as they emerge from their foramina. Branches of the two nerves are seen joining in the region of the canine, forming the so-called inner nerve loop.

PREPARATION OF THE PATIENT. The positioning of the patient and the preparation of the tissues for injection are described on page 36.

THE INJECTION. Place the bevel of the needle flat against the mucosa distal to the first molar and midway between the gingival margin and the roof of the mouth. The syringe is parallel to the sagittal plane of the molar and points somewhat distally as shown in Figure 4–13. Inform the patient that he will feel pressure as the bevel of the needle is applied against the mucosa. Enough pressure is applied so that the needle is slightly bowed. Slowly press the plunger of the syringe to force the solution against the epithelium. When blanching is observed, let the needle straighten and thus penetrate the epithelium; stop, and inject a drop of the solution. Wait 4 or 5 seconds, advance the needle a few millimeters and again stop and inject a drop. Proceed in this way until the needle has penetrated underneath the hard fibrous tissue which covers the funnel-like depression in the hard palate. This funnel-like depression is filled with loose areolar tissue and also contains the nerve and blood vessels. When the solution is injected into the space, no resistance is felt and it will readily diffuse distally. Inject no more than 0.5 ml. The method generally does not anesthetize the middle and posterior palatine nerves which supply the soft palate. Anesthetizing them gives an unpleasant sensation and should be avoided.

Nasopalatine Nerve. The bevel of the needle is placed flat against the mucosa and on the side of the incisive papilla and the bevel is pressed against the mucosa. The solution is forced against the epithelium into which it rapidly diffuses, blanching the tissues. Advance the needle barely through the epithelium and inject a drop of solution. After a pause of a few seconds direct the needle underneath the papilla and slowly inject 0.25 to 0.5 ml of the solution. The point of the needle is now under the papilla and at the entrance of the foramen. Both the right and left nasopalatine nerves will be

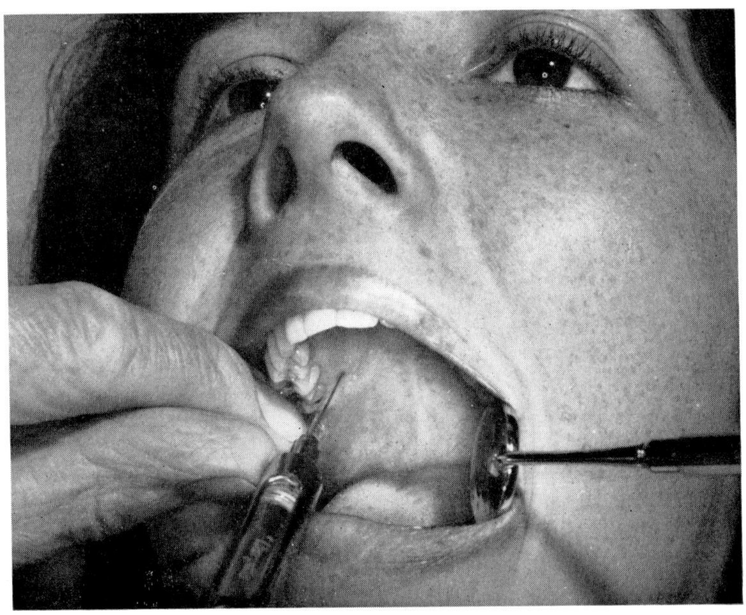

FIG. 4–13. The greater palatine nerve block.

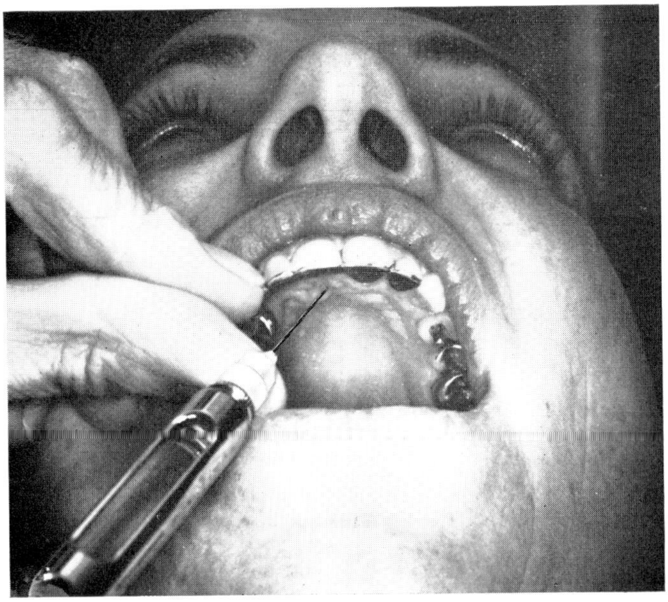

FIG. 4–14. Nasopalatine nerve block.

affected. For particularly long procedures it may be advisable to inject the solution into the canal (Fig. 4–14).

Cautions

Do not advance the needle more than 0.5 cm into the incisive canal. If the floor of the nose is entered, infection may follow.

Both the greater palatine and nasopalatine injections are generally considered to be painful procedures. The anesthetist, by skill and self-discipline, can administer the injections painlessly.

Always practice aspiration and inject slowly in minimal volumes.

The Infraorbital Nerve Block

Purpose

The infraorbital injection is the method of choice for the removal of impacted canines or large cysts, or in patients having moderate inflammation or infection which contraindicates the supraperiosteal injection. If the cellulitis is widespread, the maxillary nerve block may be chosen.

The infraorbital nerve block is effective for children's restorative and surgical dental treatment.

Failures in the supraperiosteal technique prevent adequate profundity or duration of anesthesia. If the maxillary cortical bone is smooth and dense and the molar teeth have thick bone covering the apical areas (Figs. 4–3 and 4–6), other techniques must be substituted for the supraperiosteal one.

For the upper jaw and teeth, three nerve blocks are available: (1) the infraorbital, also called the anterior infraorbital block, for the anterior and middle superior alveolar nerves; (2) the tuberosity injection for the posterior superior alveolar nerves; and (3) the maxillary nerve block, also called the posterior infraorbital block according to where it is administered. The infraorbital block will now be described.

Technique

Adult. MORPHOLOGY. The infraorbital foramen is in line with the axis of the second premolar and this axial line extends through the supraorbital notch (Figs. 4–15 and 4–18). There are rarely deviations from this rule. Observe that the foramen lies directly below the suture between the maxillary and the zygomatic bone. The foramen usually lies at the meeting point of the second and third fifths of the infraorbital margin. Finally, when the patient looks straight forward the foramen is, as a rule, 1 to 4 mm medial to the pupil of the eye (Fig. 4–16) and about 1 cm below the infraorbital margin (Fig. 4–15). The injection anesthetizes the incisors, canine and premolar teeth and their periodontium, except the palatal gingivae. Obviously, the facial tissues supplied by the cutaneous terminals of the infraorbital nerve will be affected. Anesthesia of the premolars in those patients in whom the middle superior alveolar nerve is missing is probably due to posterior flow of the solution if the injection is administered as described below. In these instances the branch from the posterior superior alveolar nerve follows the infraorbital groove for some distance before entering the lateral wall of the antrum.

Preparation of the Patient. The positioning of the patient and the preparation of the tissues for injection are described on page 36.

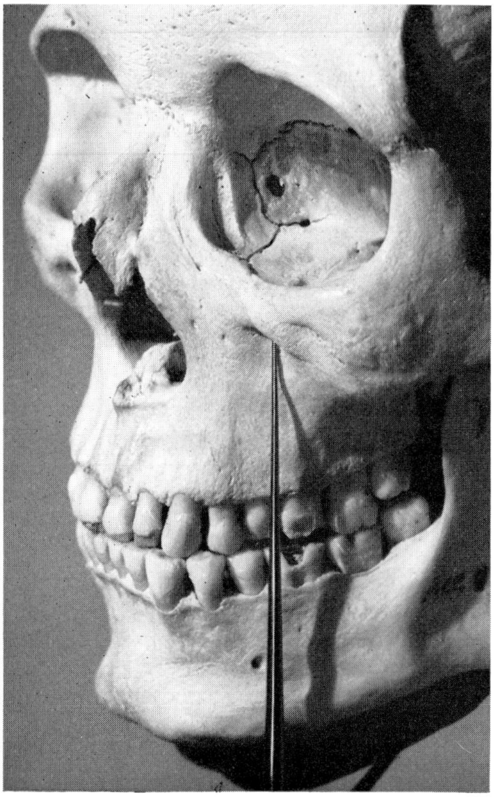

Fig. 4–15. A safe approach to the infraorbital canal along the axis of the second premolar.

The Injection. Deliberately locate the foramen, using one or more of the described methods (Fig. 4–16*A*). Place the bulb of the forefinger gently over the foramen. Use the thumb to lift the lip and cheek upward and outward. Hold the syringe in a pen grasp, placing it so that the needle is parallel with the axis of the second premolar. The barrel of the syringe lies gently against the lower lip. Insert the needle so that in spanning the infraorbital fossa its point is aimed toward the fingertip (Fig. 4–16*B*). The moment the needle point penetrates the mucosa inject a drop of the anesthetic solution, wait about 4 to 5 seconds and again gently advance the needle. As the needle penetrates the fatty areolar tissue between the levator labii superioris muscle and the levator anguli oris muscle (Fig. 4–17), there usually is little sensation. If the patient evidences discomfort, stop, inject a minim or two and wait a few seconds for anesthesia. As the needle approaches the area deep to the anesthetist's fingertip a few minims of the solution should be injected. The resultant welling in the tissues can be felt by the fingertip. Wait about 10 seconds for anesthesia of the periosteum at the foramen, then advance the needle gently past the lower border of the infraorbital foramen into the anterior part of the infraorbital canal. Apply firm pressure over the foramen with the fingertip and inject the solution slowly (Fig. 4–16*C*). The solution flows readily if the needle is in the canal and no welling in the tissues can be felt by the fingertip. Examine a skull and note that the volume of space provided by the groove and the canal is not large enough to contain 2 ml of solution.

Furthermore, in a patient the space available for solution is reduced by the presence of a neurovascular bundle. The rule is to inject 0.5 to 0.75 ml into the canal over a period of two minutes. The injection is extremely simple to master. From the beginning it can be ascertained if the needle is in the canal. The several thousand infraorbital injections given by sophomore, junior, and senior dental students at the Loma Linda University School of Dentistry have not resulted in hematomas or other unpleasant or serious side effects.

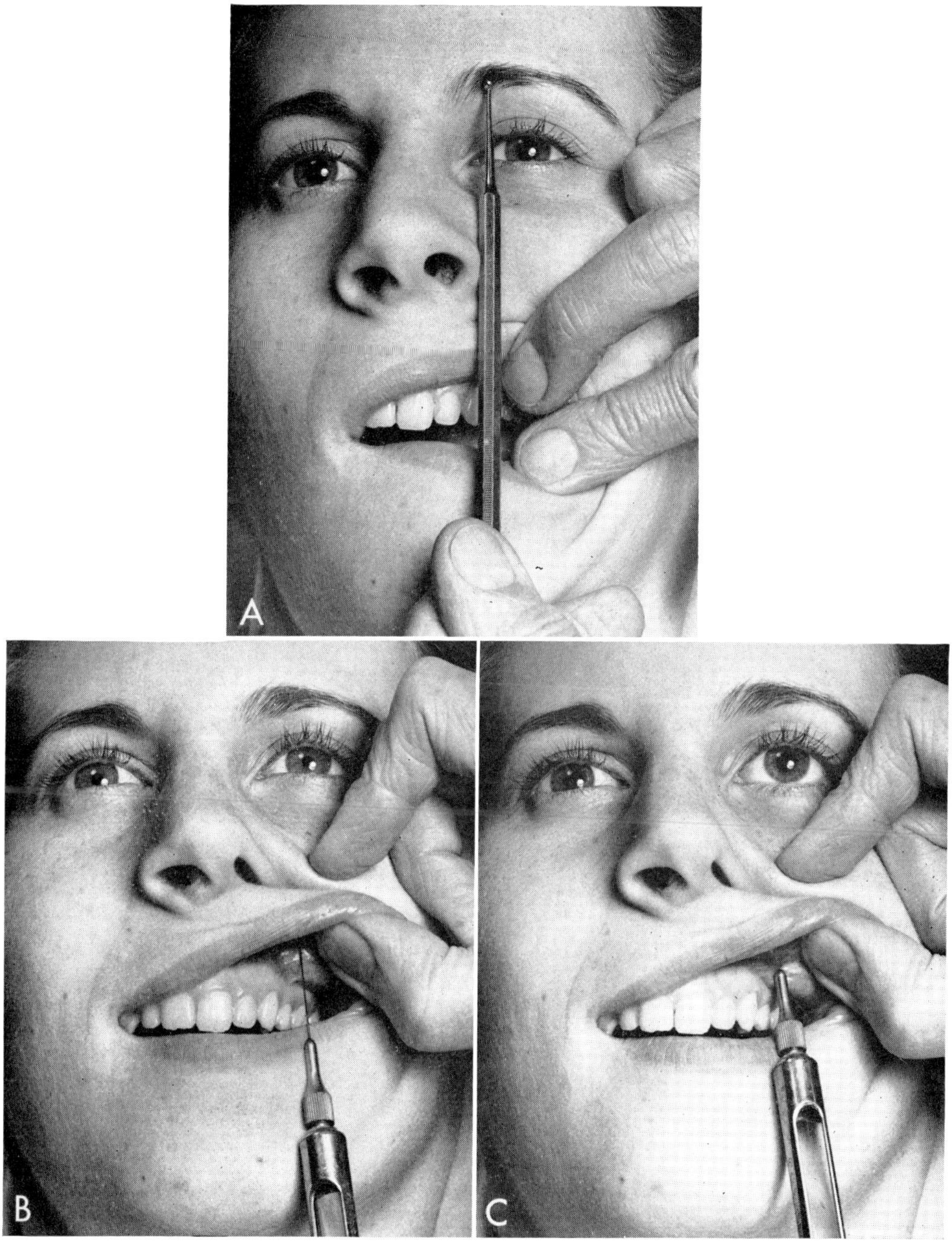

FIG. 4–16. Oblique views. *A*, Demonstrating the relationship of the supraorbital notch, infraorbital foramen and the second premolar. *B*, Aiming the needle toward the infraorbital foramen. *C*, Needle in foramen.

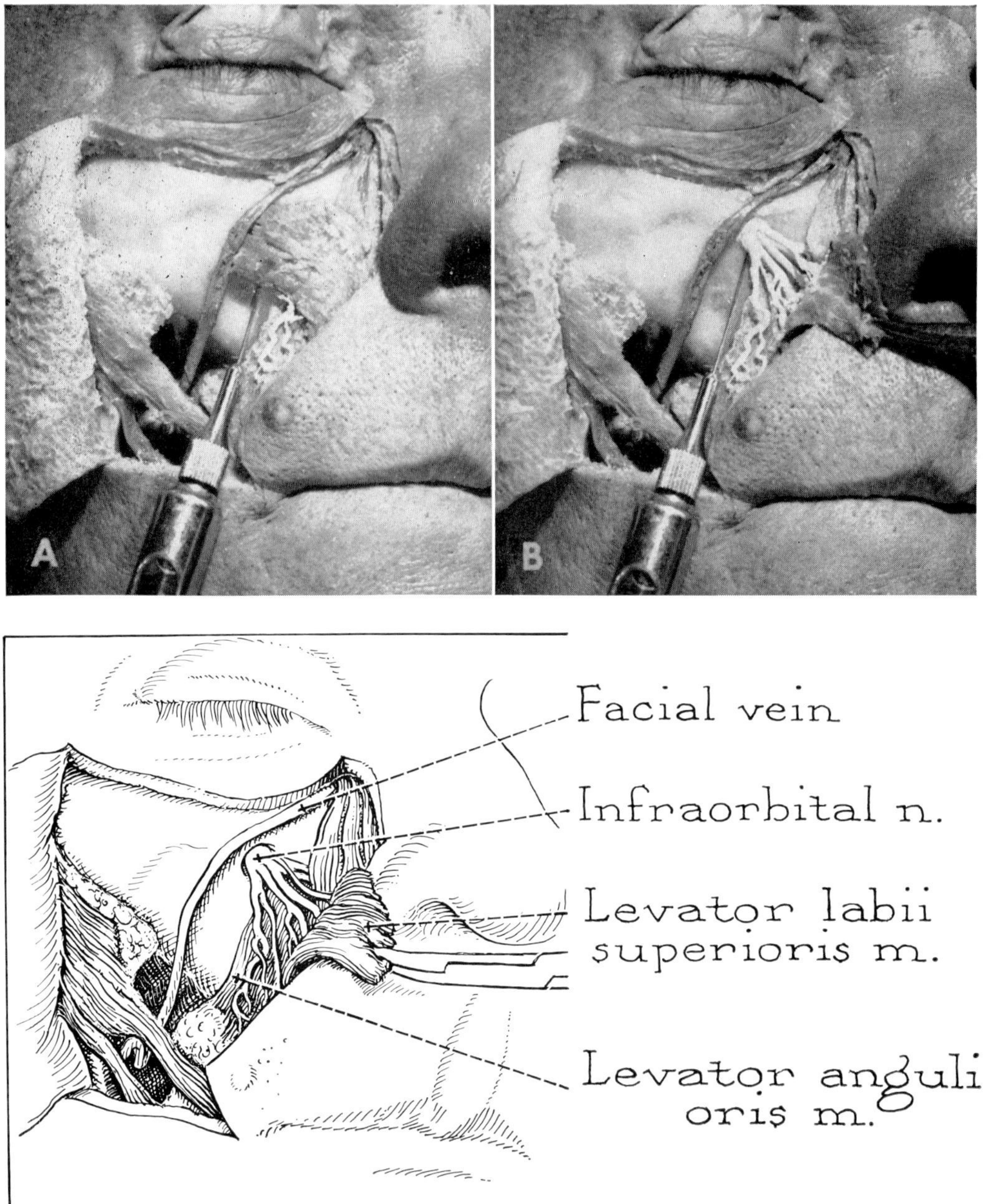

FIG. 4–17. *A*, The relation of the needle to the levator labii superioris and levator anguli oris muscles in the canine fossa. *B*, The levator labii retracted.

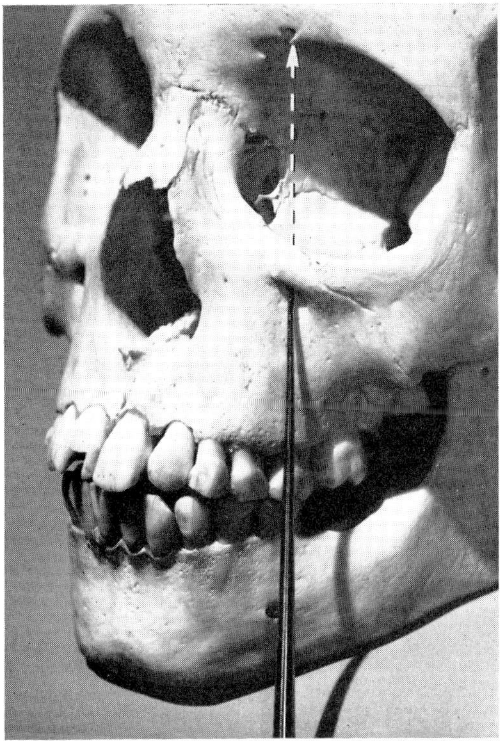

FIG. 4–18. Classic relation of supraorbital notch, zygomaticomaxillary suture, and infraorbital and mental foramina.

Child. The depth of needle penetration for the infraorbital injections in a child is little more than for the supraperiosteal injection because of the low height of the maxilla (Fig. 4–18). It will be recalled that to affect the primary molars the supraperiosteal injection is given high on the lateral wall of the antrum.

Cautions

Some individuals deposit the solution in the region of the infraorbital foramen and then, with massage, "force the solution" into the infraorbital canal. Experience indicates that this method seldom gives proper pulpal anesthesia. Because the anterior superior alveolar nerves leave the infraorbital nerve 7 to 10 mm posterior to the foramen, others advise that the needle be introduced this distance into the canal. The syringe then lies over the central incisors and the needle enters the canal in a posterior lateral direction. For the inexperienced there is danger that the needle may enter the eyeball (Fig. 4–19).

Always practice aspiration and inject slowly in minimal volumes.

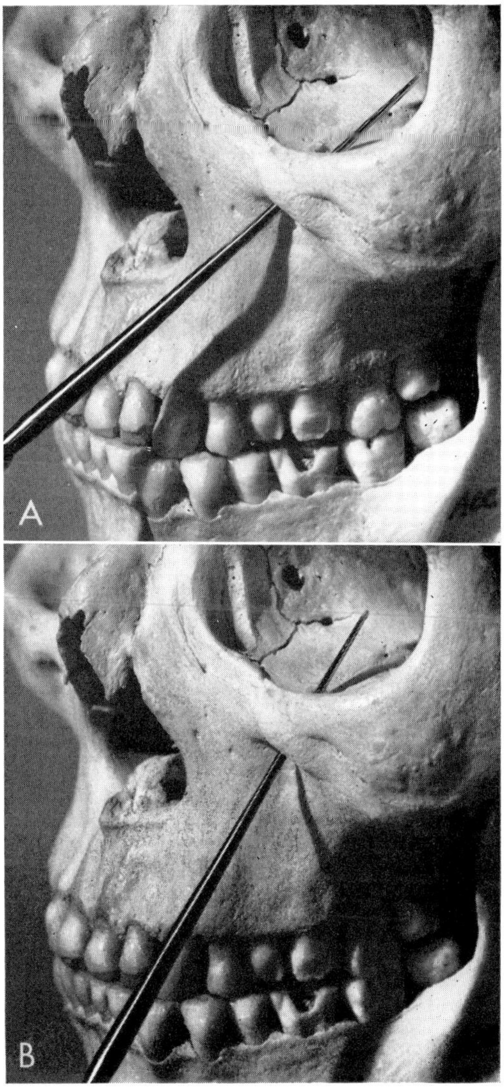

FIG. 4–19. Two possibilities for entering the orbit when using the direct approach to the infraorbital canal. *A*, Path from maxillary central incisors to foramen. *B*, Failure to keep close to lower lip.

The Posterior Superior Alveolar Nerve Block (Tuberosity)

Purpose

The tuberosity, or zygomatic, block is the simplest method to obtain immediate anesthesia of the posterior superior alveolar nerves. It produces profound pulpal and surgical anesthesia where the supraperiosteal technique may fail. The tuberosity injection is also indicated in certain cases if infection or inflammation contraindicates a supraperiosteal injection.

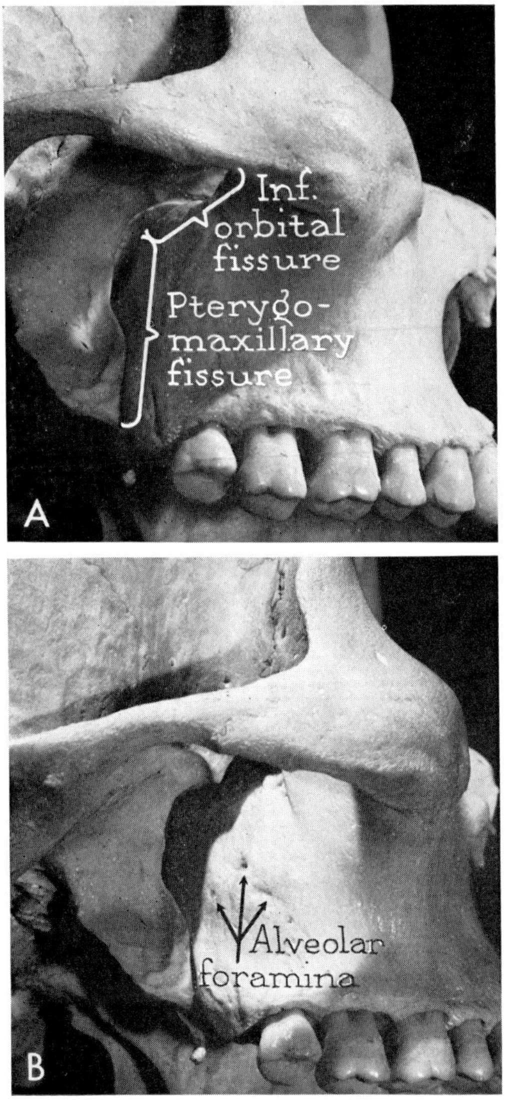

FIG. 4–20. The maxilla. *A*, Posterior relations. *B*, Alveolar foramina on the tuberosity.

Technique

Straight Hub Needle. MORPHOLOGY. From Figure 4–20 it can be observed that the foramina for the posterior superior alveolar nerves are located midway between the upper and lower posterior part of the maxilla and a few millimeters medial to the most prominent part of the tuberosity when viewed in three-quarter profile. On Figures 4–3 and 4–7 notice that the height of the maxilla may vary considerably. The range of measurements of several hundred skulls* varied from 27 to 66 mm on adults' skulls with the teeth in occlusion. The anterior and posterior heights of the maxilla are the same (Fig. 4–21*A* and *B*). The anterior height of the maxilla can be ascertained by using a Boley gauge to measure the distance from the infraorbital margin to the gingiva of the premolars (Fig. 4–22). Figure 4–23 demonstrates the posterior superior alveolar nerve's straight course downward on the periosteum from the maxillary nerve to the foramina. Notice the other soft structures in the infratemporal fossa, such as the maxillary artery on the lateral surface of the lateral pterygoid muscle. The pterygoid plexus of veins and the fat pad were removed.

PREPARATION OF THE PATIENT. The positioning of the patient and the preparation of the tissues for injection are described on page 36.

THE INJECTION. While cleansing the oral mucosa, find the spot for the needle insertion by ascertaining where the cotton applicator slides upward distal to the zygomatic process of the maxilla. The patient's mouth is only slightly open and the patient is instructed to move the lower jaw toward the side of the injection. Obviously, this allows more space for the manipulation of the syringe between the coronoid process and the maxilla. The cheek is stretched upward and outward with the thumb, the needle inserted through the movable mucosa and a drop of the solution injected. After 4 or 5 seconds the

* Now at University of Pacific, Atkinson Collection.

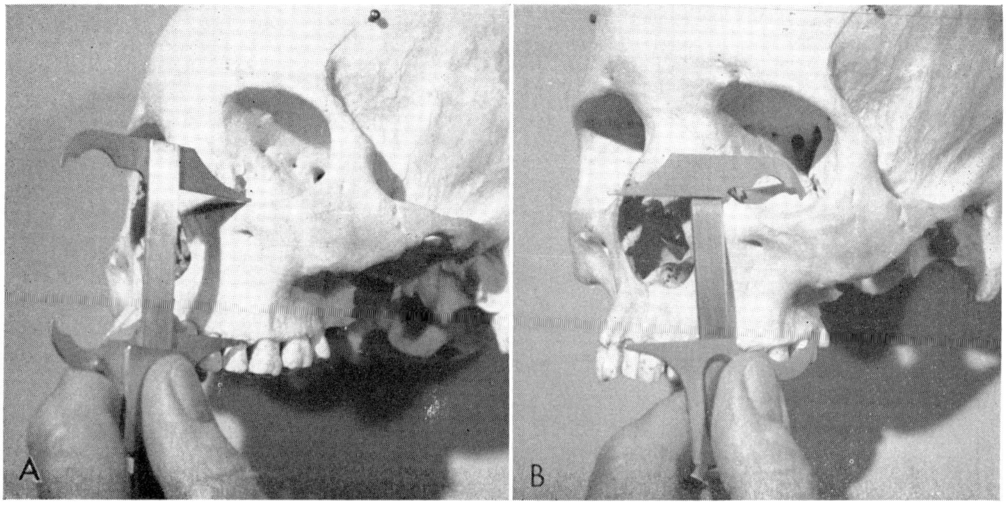

FIG. 4–21. Measuring the maxillary height. *A*, Anterior. *B*, Posterior.

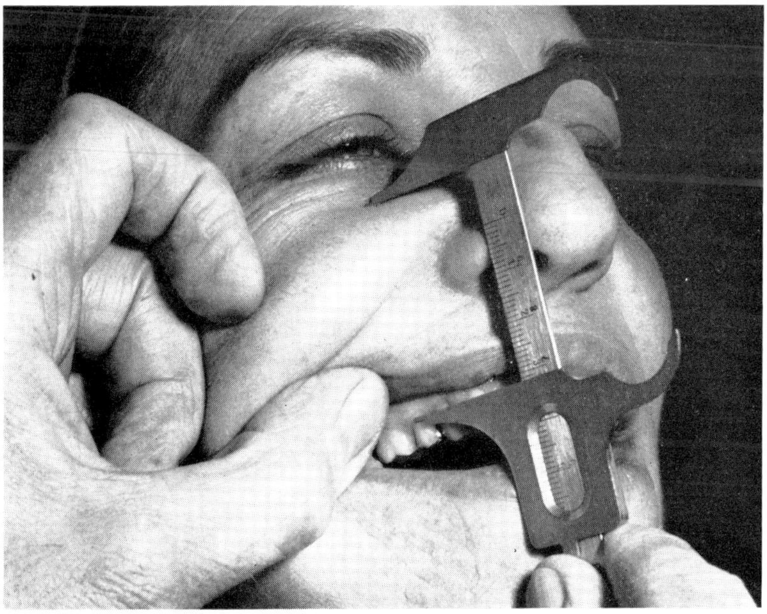

FIG. 4–22. Measuring the anterior maxillary height.

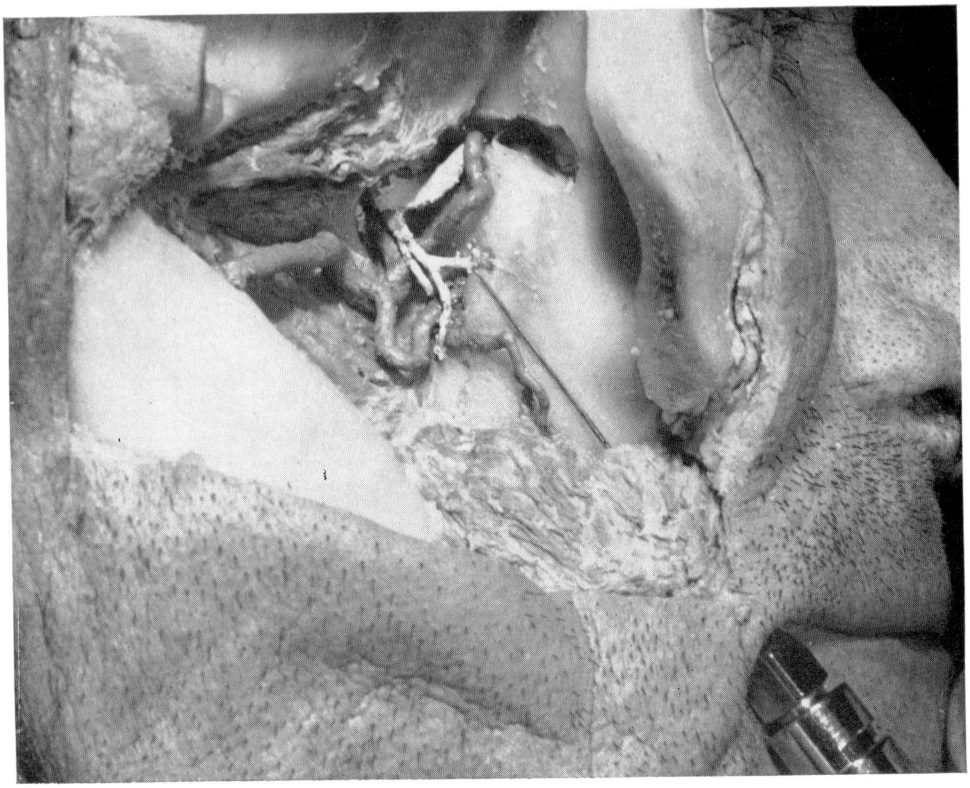

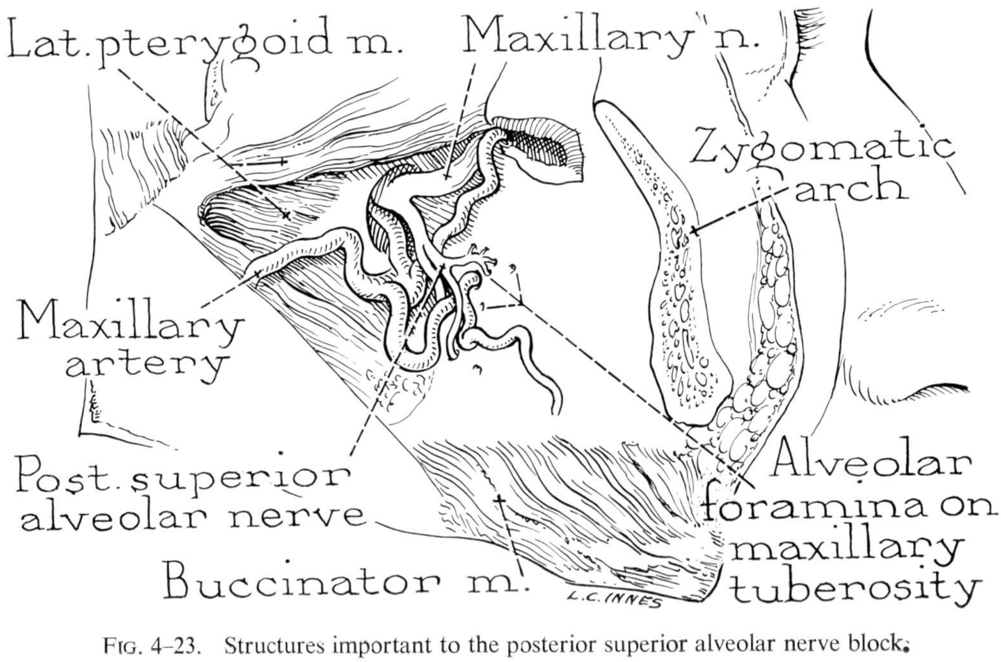

FIG. 4-23. Structures important to the posterior superior alveolar nerve block.

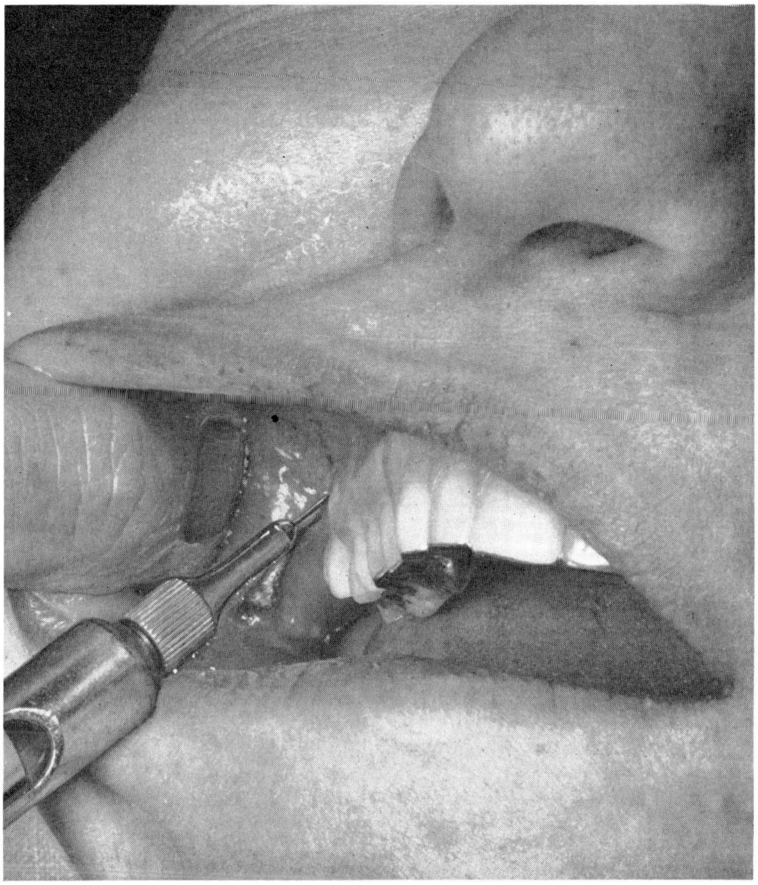

FIG. 4–24. The posterior superior alveolar nerve block.

needle is advanced a few millimeters upward, inward and backward and a drop is injected before the periosteum is touched. Proceed by steps. As the needle slides along the periosteum, inject a drop of the solution at each step. Stop, aspirate and inject from 0.5 to 1 ml of the solution the moment the needle loses contact with the curvature of the tuberosity (Fig. 4–24).

For the median maxillary height, the angulation of the needle relative to both the occlusal and the sagittal planes is 45 degrees. In a high maxilla, the angulation of the needle is greater, up to 70 degrees. In the low maxilla of some adults and most children, the angulation lies between 20 and 30 degrees.

Bent Hub Needle. Considering all the dimensional variations, the bent hub needle provides the simpler and more accurate technique.[5] The point of needle insertion is opposite the third molar. The needle is advanced by steps, but only until the midpoint of the height of the maxilla has been reached where, after aspiration, 0.25 to 0.5 ml is injected. To determine accurately the precise location for the needle tip at the moment of injection, fix a small piece of sterile rubber dam (placed prior to sterilization of the needle) on the needle at a distance from the tip of the needle of one half of the measured maxillary height (compare with Fig. 4–22).

Cautions

The angulation of insertion is important because a misdirected needle tip can cause injury. If the penetration is relatively too deep (high), the maxillary artery is often injured. When the needle does not deviate sufficiently from the sagittal plane, the pterygoid plexus of veins or the lateral pterygoid muscle is injured (Fig. 4–23).

In some cases, complete anesthesia will not be present in the maxillary first permanent molar because fibers from the middle superior alveolar nerve innervate the mesiobuccal root of this tooth. In these cases the supraperiosteal injection is given anterior to the zygomatic process of the maxilla.

Always practice aspiration and inject slowly, in minimal volumes.

The Maxillary Nerve Block

Purpose

At times it is advantageous, for diagnostic block and for extensive surgery of the upper jaw and teeth, to block the maxillary nerve itself rather than its peripheral branches. This is also indicated when inflammation or infection precludes the more peripheral approaches. Furthermore, the anesthetic solution should be deposited at, or near, the nerve as it courses across the pterygopalatine fossa.

Arthur Smith's[13] technique is the simplest, and provides the safest approach. The needle approaches anteriorly to the maxillary artery (Fig. 4–23).

Technique

Lateral Approach. MORPHOLOGY. For this injection the anesthetist does not have definite bony landmarks to determine the proper depth for the needle insertion. From Figures 4–3 and 4–7 it can be observed that the height of the maxilla varies greatly, but the posterior height of the maxilla can be ascertained simply by measuring the height of the maxilla from the infraorbital margin to the gingiva of the premolars.[6] This height has been found to be the same as the posterior height of the maxilla (Fig. 4–25).

PREPARATION OF THE PATIENT. The positioning of the patient and the preparation of the tissues for injection are described on page 36.

THE INJECTION. A Boley gauge is used to obtain the height of the maxilla (Fig. 4–25*A*). A bent needle, or a straight needle in a bent hub, is used. A sterile piece of rubber placed on the needle serves as a marker which is adjusted to show the measured maxillary height (Fig. 4–25*B*). The cheek of the patient is stretched outward and upward with the operator's first finger, and the patient is asked to open the jaw and move it toward the side of the intended injection. The

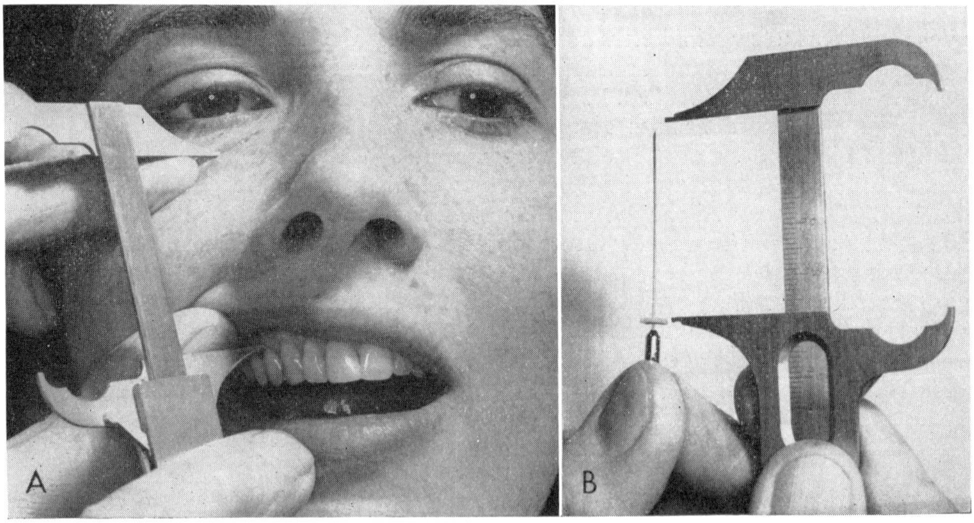

FIG. 4–25. *A*, Measuring the maxillary height. *B*, Adjusting the marker to correspond to the measured maxillary height.

needle is inserted at the height of the vestibule, generally opposite the last molar and some distance from the alveolar mucosa, and directed upward, inward and backward (Fig. 4–26*A*). The needle should not touch the periosteum until it has penetrated 15 mm (Fig. 4–26*B*). Before it touches the periosteum, 2 drops of the solution are injected. A few seconds are allowed to elapse before the needle is advanced along the periosteum and a small amount of the solution is again injected. After another few seconds have

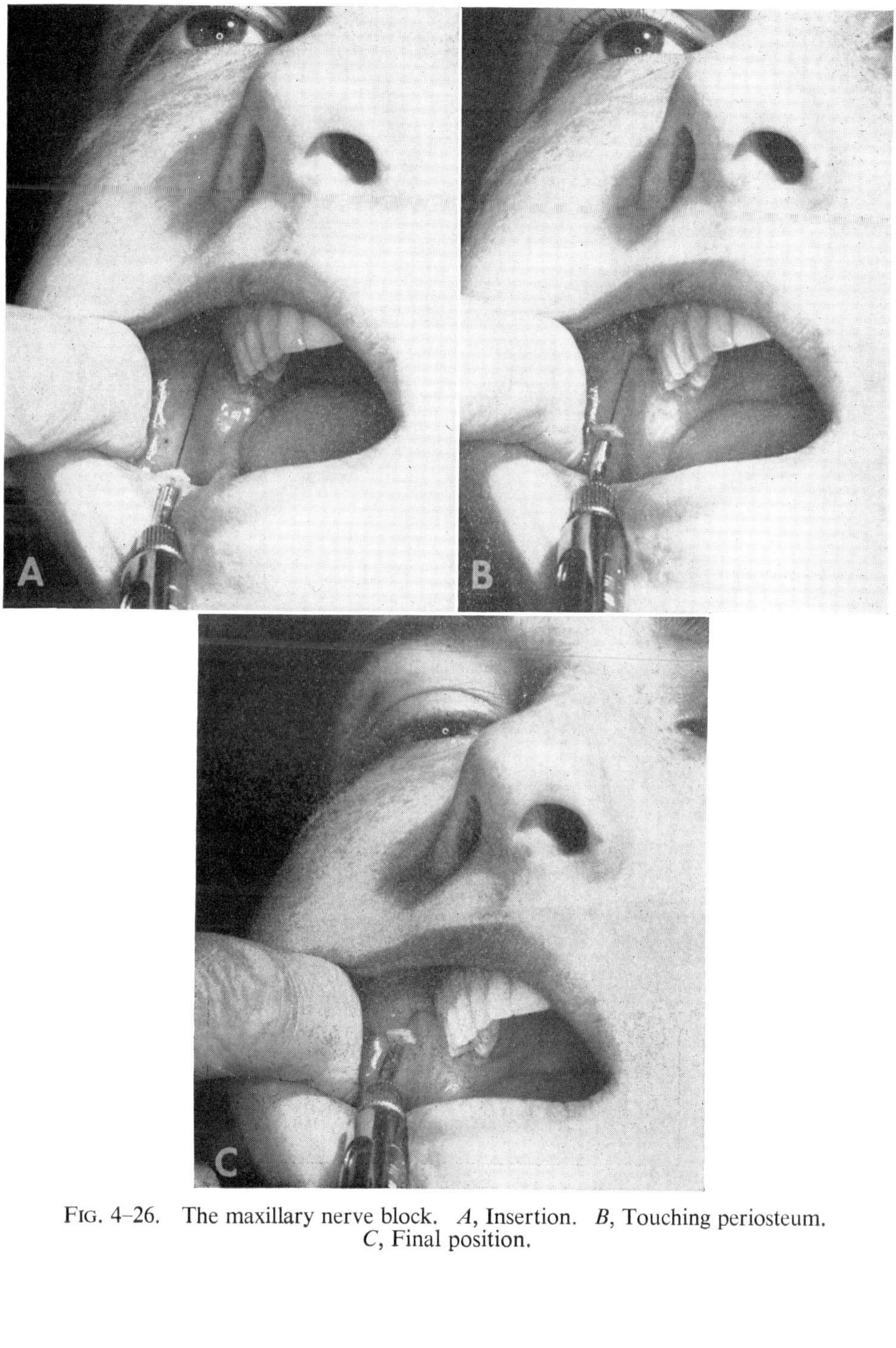

FIG. 4–26. The maxillary nerve block. *A*, Insertion. *B*, Touching periosteum. *C*, Final position.

elapsed, the needle is again advanced and a small amount of solution injected. This method permits the injection to be painless and without proprioceptive sensation. The needle is advanced until the rubber marker is in line with a horizontal plane through the gingival margin of the second molar (Figs. 4–26*C* and 4–27*A*). The solution remaining in the cartridge is then injected.

Greater Palatine Canal Approach. Many anesthetists prefer to pass the needle through the greater palatine canal into the pterygopalatine fossa to block the maxillary nerve (Fig. 4–27*B* and *C*). The greater palatine foramen is easily located; it is always found in the same sagittal plane and anterior to the pterygoid hamulus and can easily be palpated with a burnisher or cotton swab. The depth of penetration is determined in the same way as for the lateral approach. If the patient cannot open his mouth wide, a needle with a bent hub should be used. The anesthetist

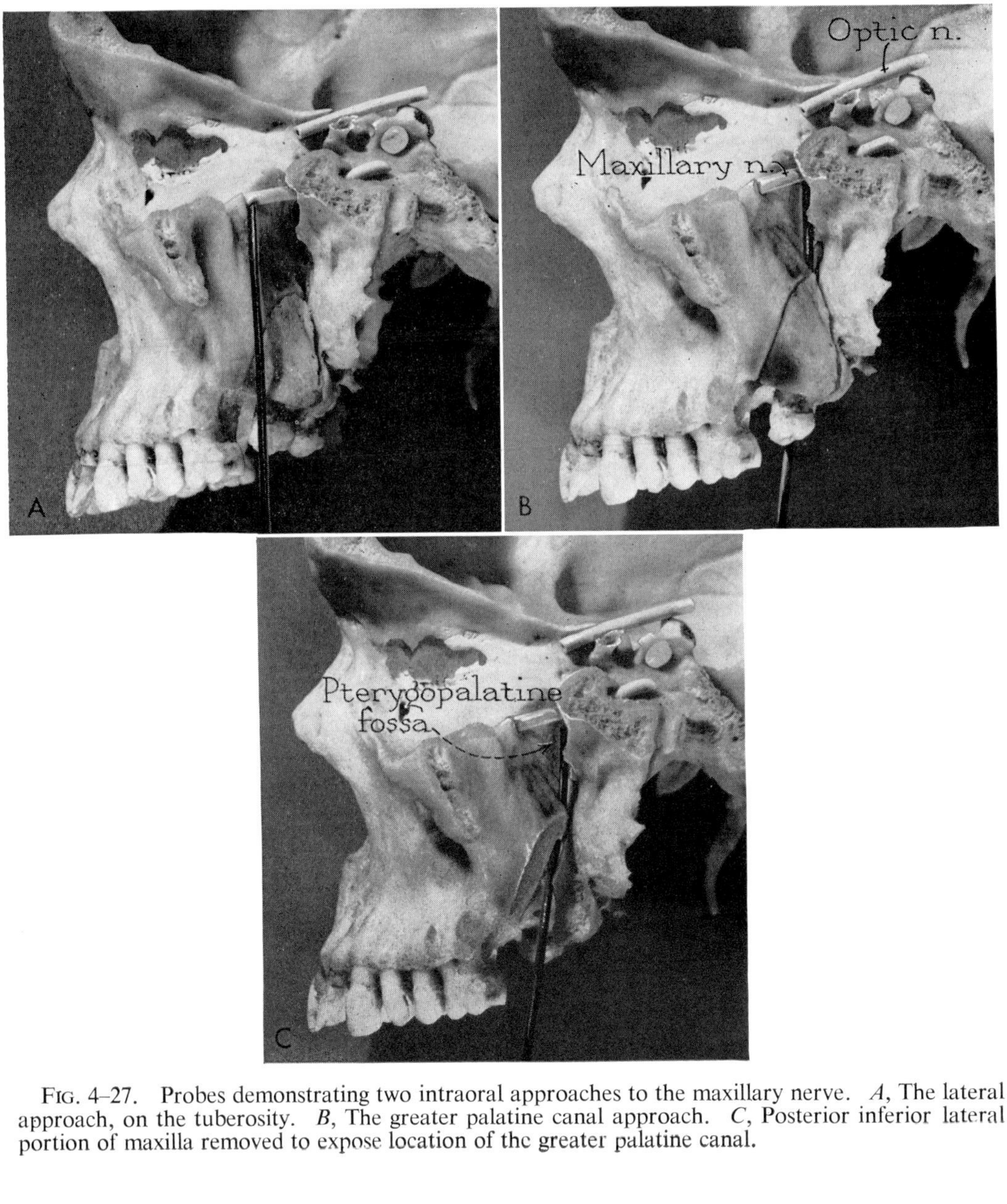

FIG. 4–27. Probes demonstrating two intraoral approaches to the maxillary nerve. *A*, The lateral approach, on the tuberosity. *B*, The greater palatine canal approach. *C*, Posterior inferior lateral portion of maxilla removed to expose location of the greater palatine canal.

must take care that the advancing needle is kept in the sagittal plane. If it deviates laterally and distally it will, in many cases, slip through the pterygomaxillary fissure into the infratemporal space (Fig. 4–28*A*). If it deviates medially it may penetrate the often paper-thin medial wall of the pterygopalatine fossa and enter the nasal space (Fig. 4–28*B*). If the needle is carried relatively too far—which can easily happen in a short skull—it will enter the orbit (Fig. 4–28*C*). It goes without saying, also, that a heavy needle, not less than 25-gauge, and with a short bevel, should be used. Extreme care must be taken in regard to asepsis when this injection is employed.

Caution

The route through the greater palatine canal does not always give unhindered access to the fossa. In probing the canal in more than 200 skulls, bony obstructions were present in 15 per cent of them.

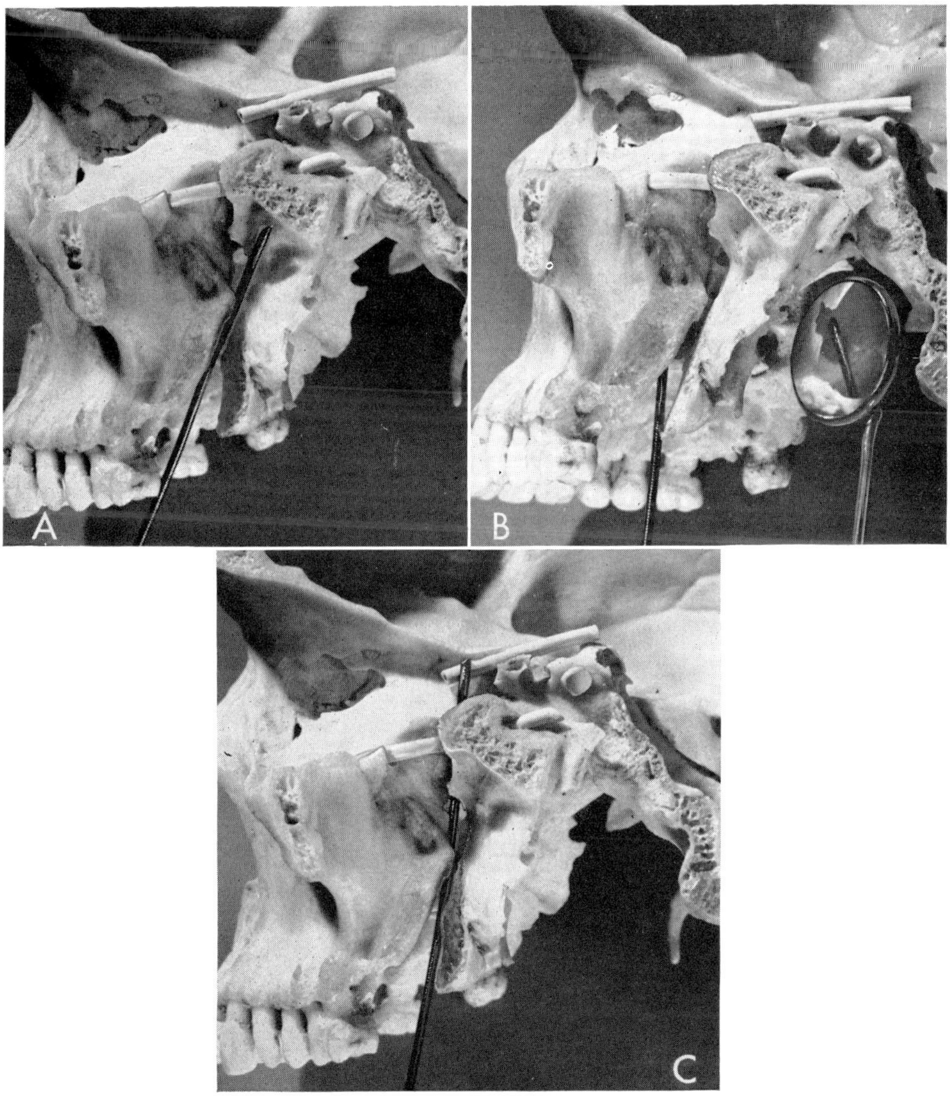

FIG. 4–28. Probes demonstrating hazards of the two intraoral approaches to the maxillary nerve. *A*, Needle in infratemporal fossa. *B*, Needle in nasal cavity. *C*, Needle in orbital cavity.

The lateral approach may be along the tuberosity of the maxilla toward the inferior orbital fissure near the entrance of the nerve into the orbit (Fig. 4–27*A*) or further medio-posteriorly so that the needle enters the fossa itself. From Figure 4–23 it is evident that this last approach is in the path of the maxillary artery; the artery can easily be punctured by the needle, causing a severe hematoma.

Always practice aspiration and inject slowly in minimal volumes.

DIMENSIONS AND STRUCTURES IMPORTANT TO ANESTHESIA OF THE INFERIOR ALVEOLAR NERVE AND ITS TERMINALS

The purpose of the following discussion is to relate the topography of the mandible to the inferior alveolar injection. Observe Figures 4–3 and 4–29 and notice that the cortical bone of the mandible, including the alveolar processes, is smooth and dense and has no small perforations as does the alveolar area of the maxilla (Figs. 4–4 and 4–20). The only exception to this rule is the area of the incisive fossa, where small nutritional canals are often present. Observe that the lower border of the mandible and the alveolar crest are approximately parallel. The narrowest anterior-posterior length of the mandibular ramus varies considerably. The coronoid notch, *i.e.*, the bottom of the concavity of the anterior border of the ramus, varies in its distance from the occlusal plane of the posterior teeth as indicated in Figure 4–30; however, observe that a plane through this point and parallel with the occlusal surface passes just above the lingula.[8] As a rule, the height of the lingula thus can be determined prior to the injection of an anesthetic solution.

The relation holds true in children's mandibles but in adult mandibles there are three exceptions: (1) In the mandible with the variance in height (Fig. 4–30*C*) it is evident that a plane through the coronoid notch parallel with the occlusal plane of the teeth will in this case lie below the lingula. Notice also that the height of the mandible at the symphysis is almost twice that in the second molar region. (2) The lingula in prognathic mandibles is always located higher than the rule would indicate, even as much as 1 cm above the plane through the coronoid notch (Figs. 4–31 and 4–32*A*). (3) In partially or totally edentulous mandibles the plane through the coronoid notch

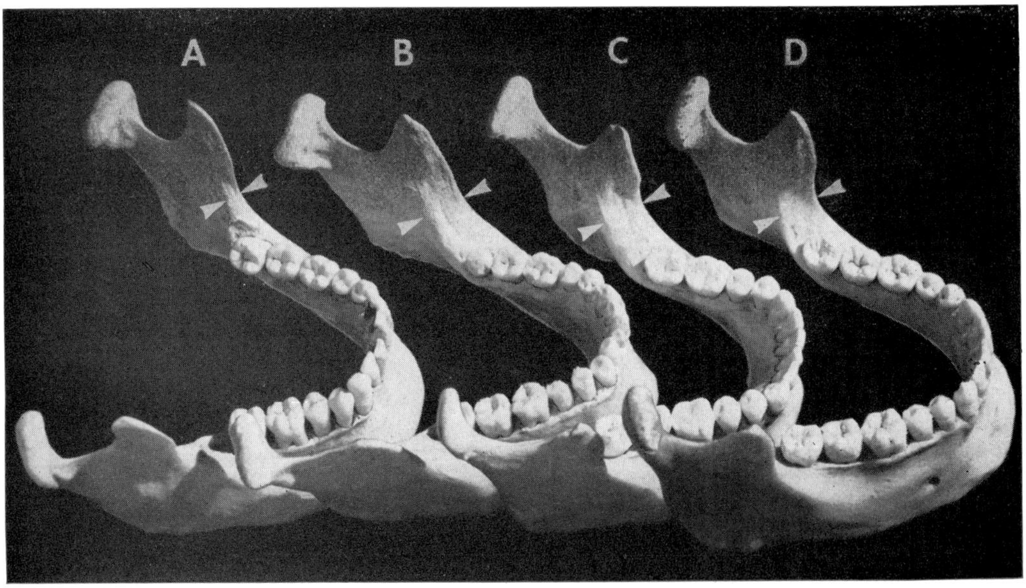

FIG. 4–29. The distance between the internal and external oblique line of the mandible varies.

must be parallel with the lower border of the mandible (Fig. 4–32*B* and *C*).

The width of the rami may vary considerably (Fig. 4–30). However, the distance from the lingula to the internal oblique line is the same (± 1 mm) irrespective of the width of the ramus or the age of the individual (compare Figs. 4–33, 4–38). Look at the ramus from the medial aspect and notice that the mandibular canal opens into a rather large, deep depression, the mandibular sulcus, overhung anteriorly by the lingula. The anterior border of the sulcus is approximately at the middle of the ramus. The anteromedial surface of the ramus is formed by the internal oblique line, or temporal crest, which is a direct continuation of the mylohyoid line (Fig. 4–33).

As explained in detail by Sicher,[11] the sulcus is the logical place to deposit the solution. The sulcus is bordered laterally by the medial surface of the ramus and medially by the medial pterygoid muscle. Since about 1 cm of the nerve lies along the anterior border of the sulcus, it would seem extremely simple to administer the injection with complete success. Obviously, the clinical facts are to the contrary. By studying the soft structures anterior and medial to the sulcus the reason may be comprehended. The sphenomandibular ligament is attached from the tip of the lingula along the anterior inferior border of the sulcus (Figs. 4–34 and 4–35). Notice that the inferior alveolar nerve lies lateral to the ligament at its anterior point.

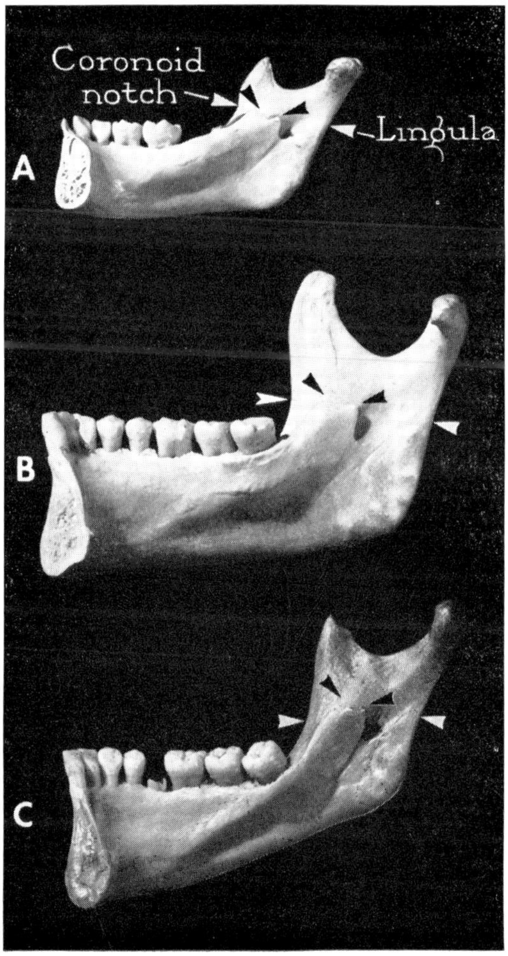

FIG. 4–30. Variations in the height of the lingula and anterior-posterior dimensions of the ramus.

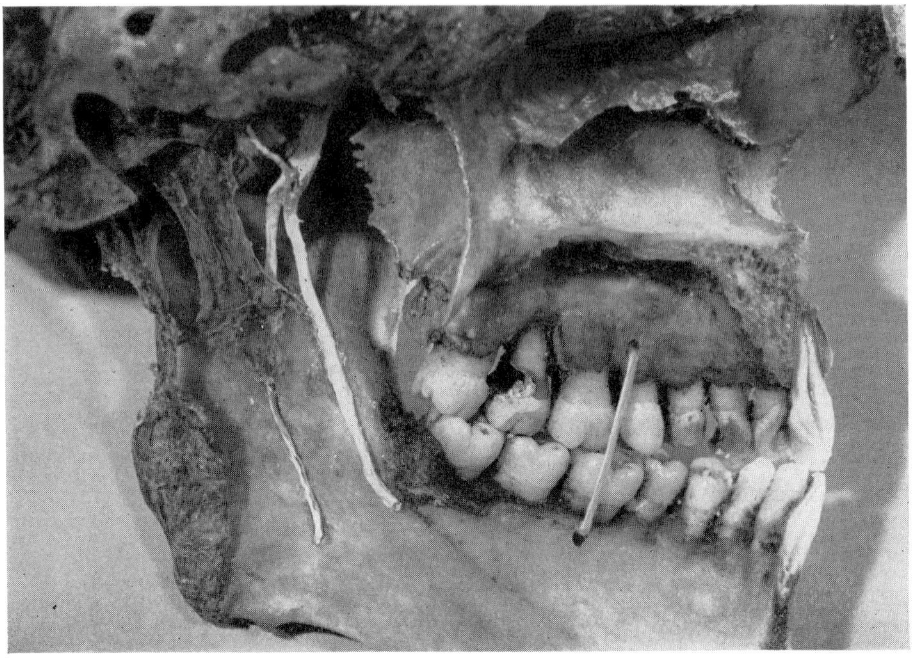

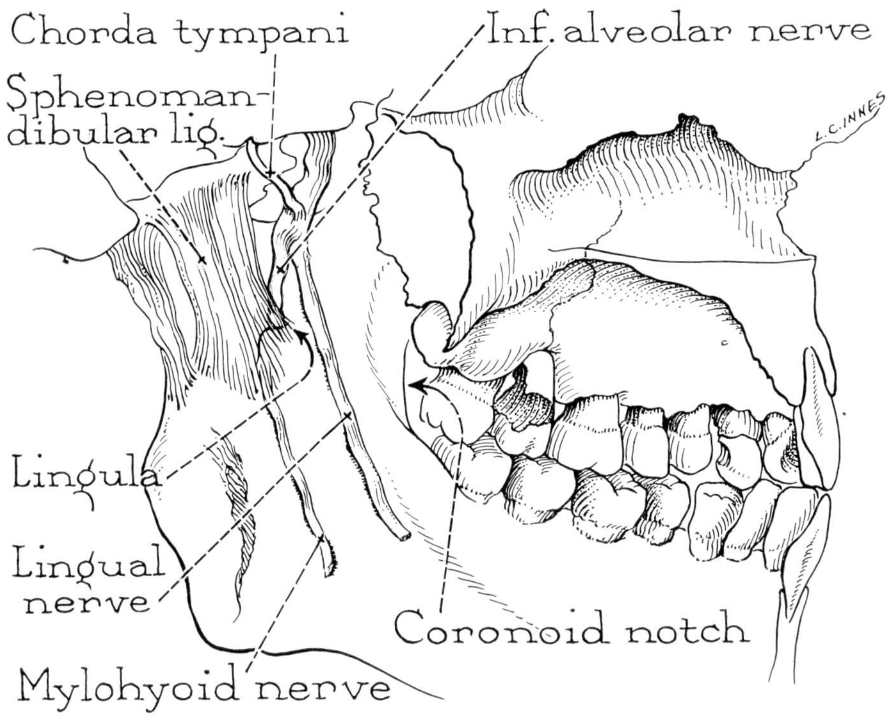

FIG. 4–31. Prognathic mandible.

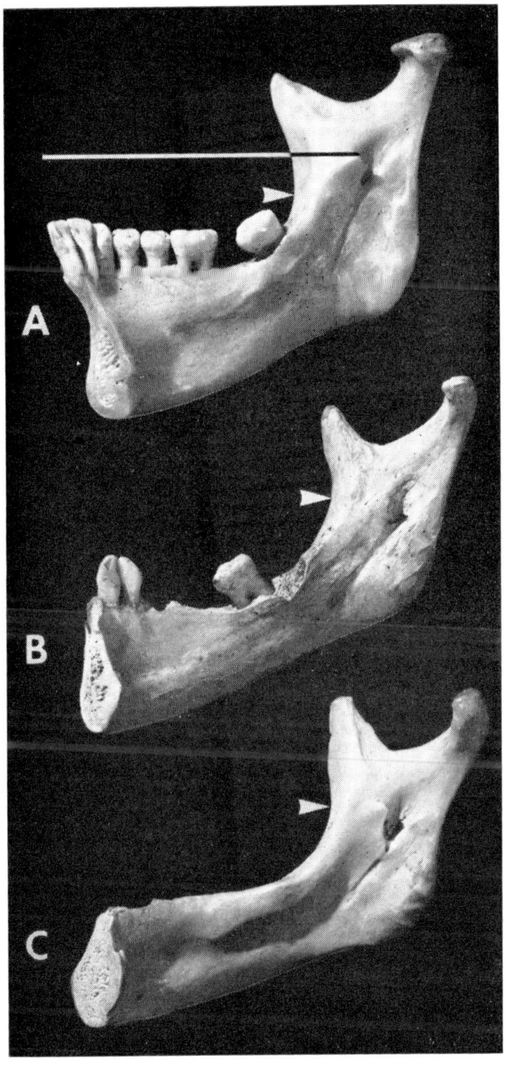

FIG. 4–32. Mandibles. *A*, Prognathic. *B*, Mutilated. *C*, Edentulous.

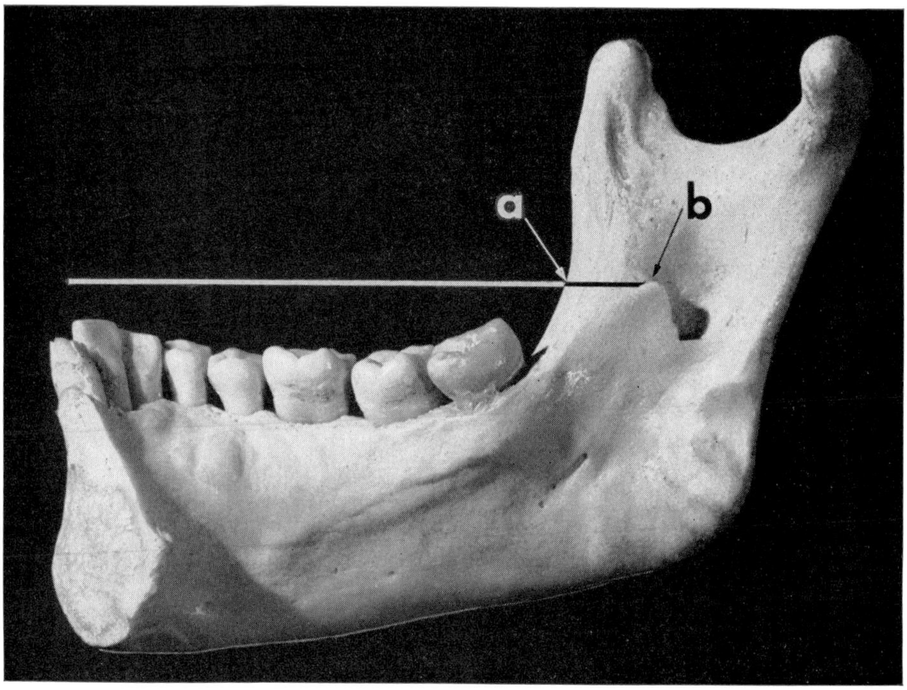

FIG. 4–33. Plane passing through coronoid notch (*a*) and above lingula (*b*).

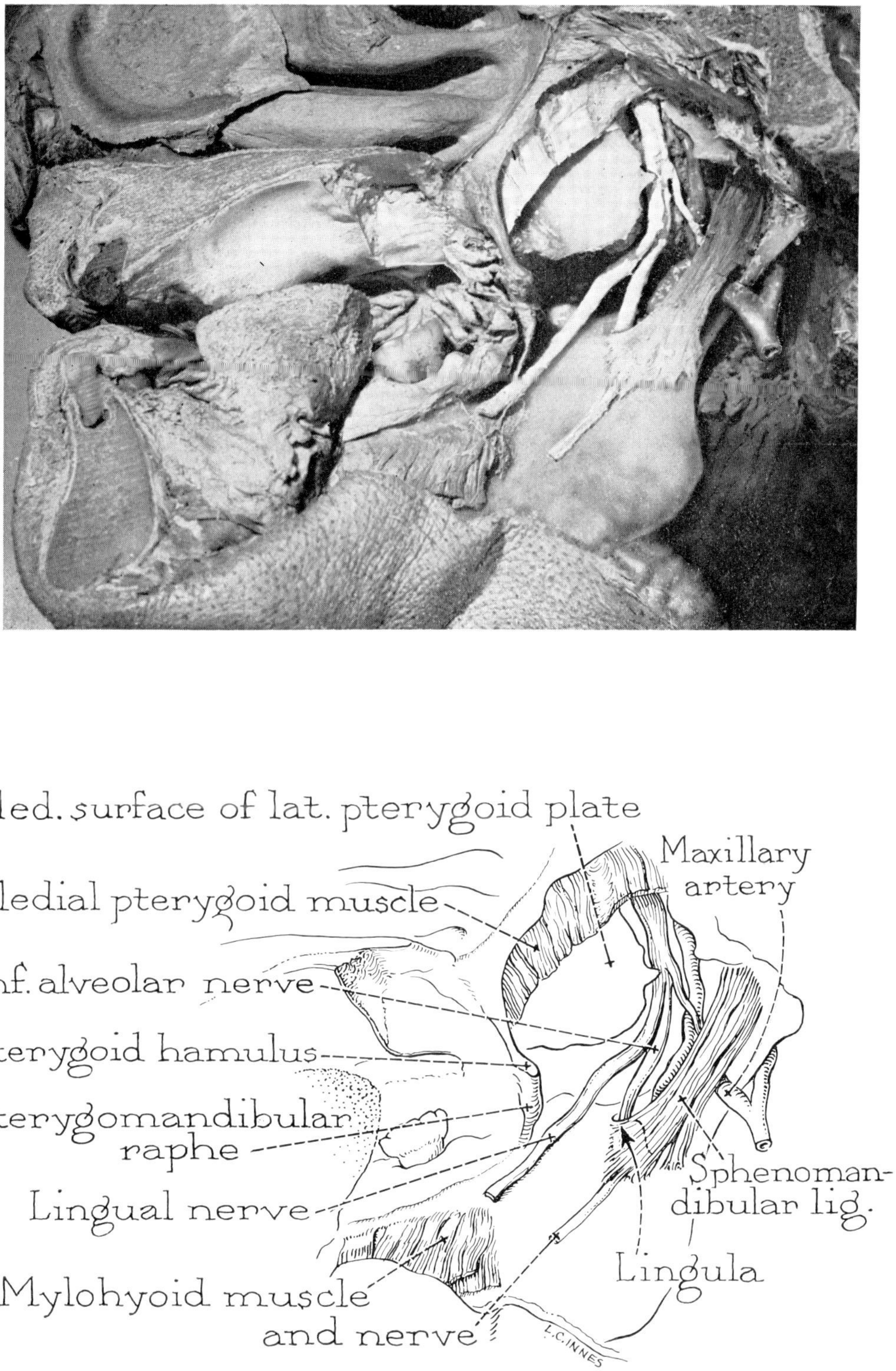

FIG. 4–34. Medial view of the pterygomandibular space.

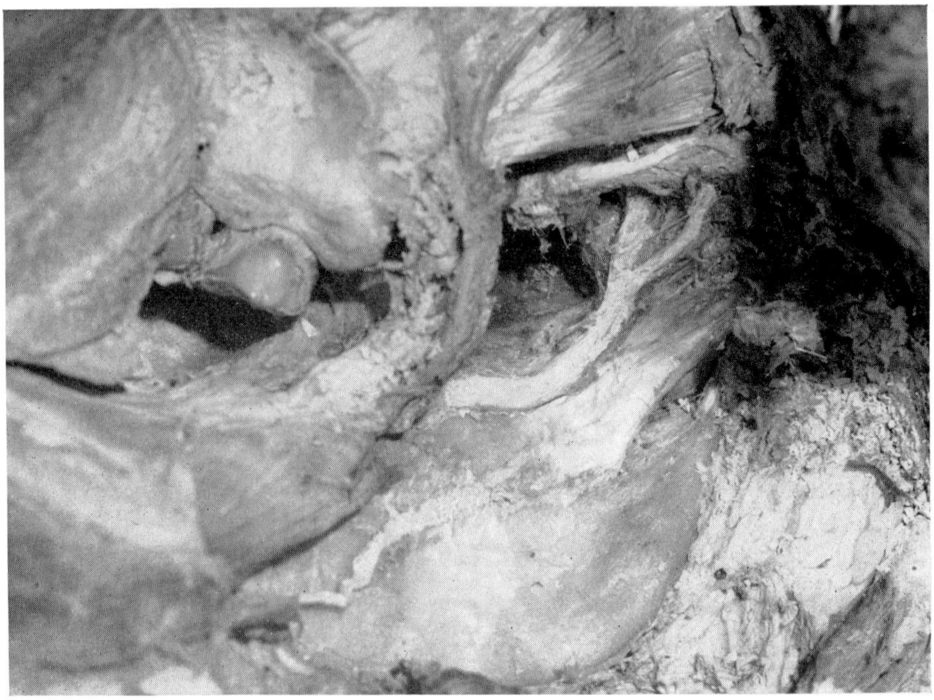

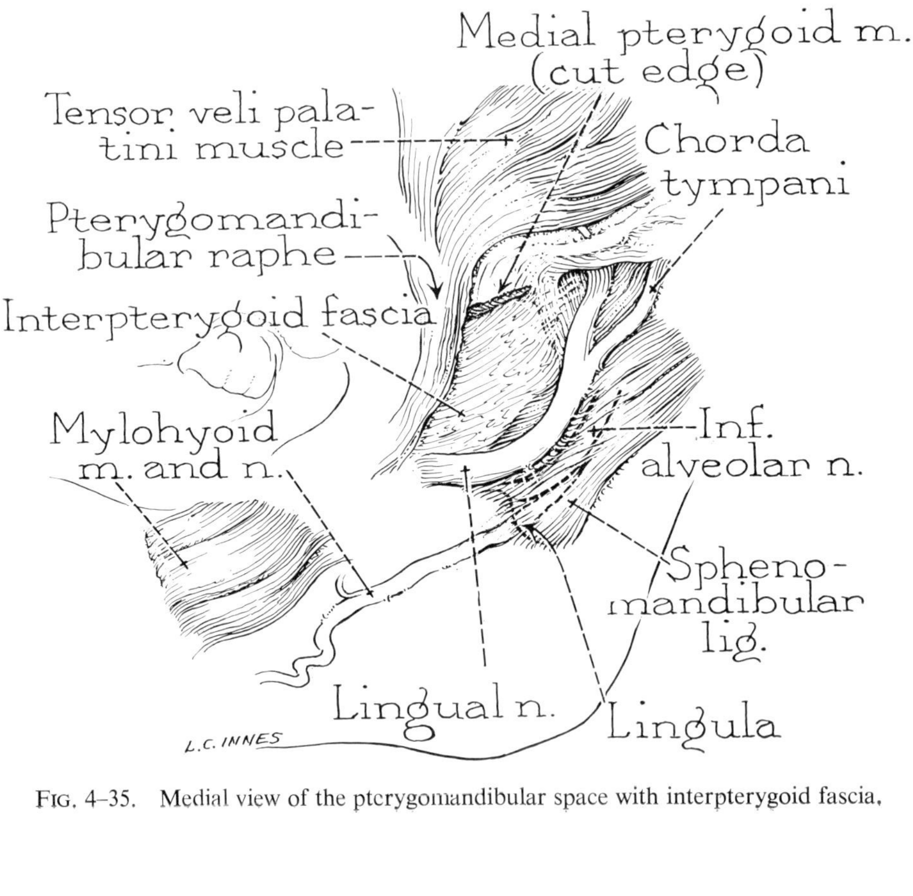

FIG. 4–35. Medial view of the pterygomandibular space with interpterygoid fascia.

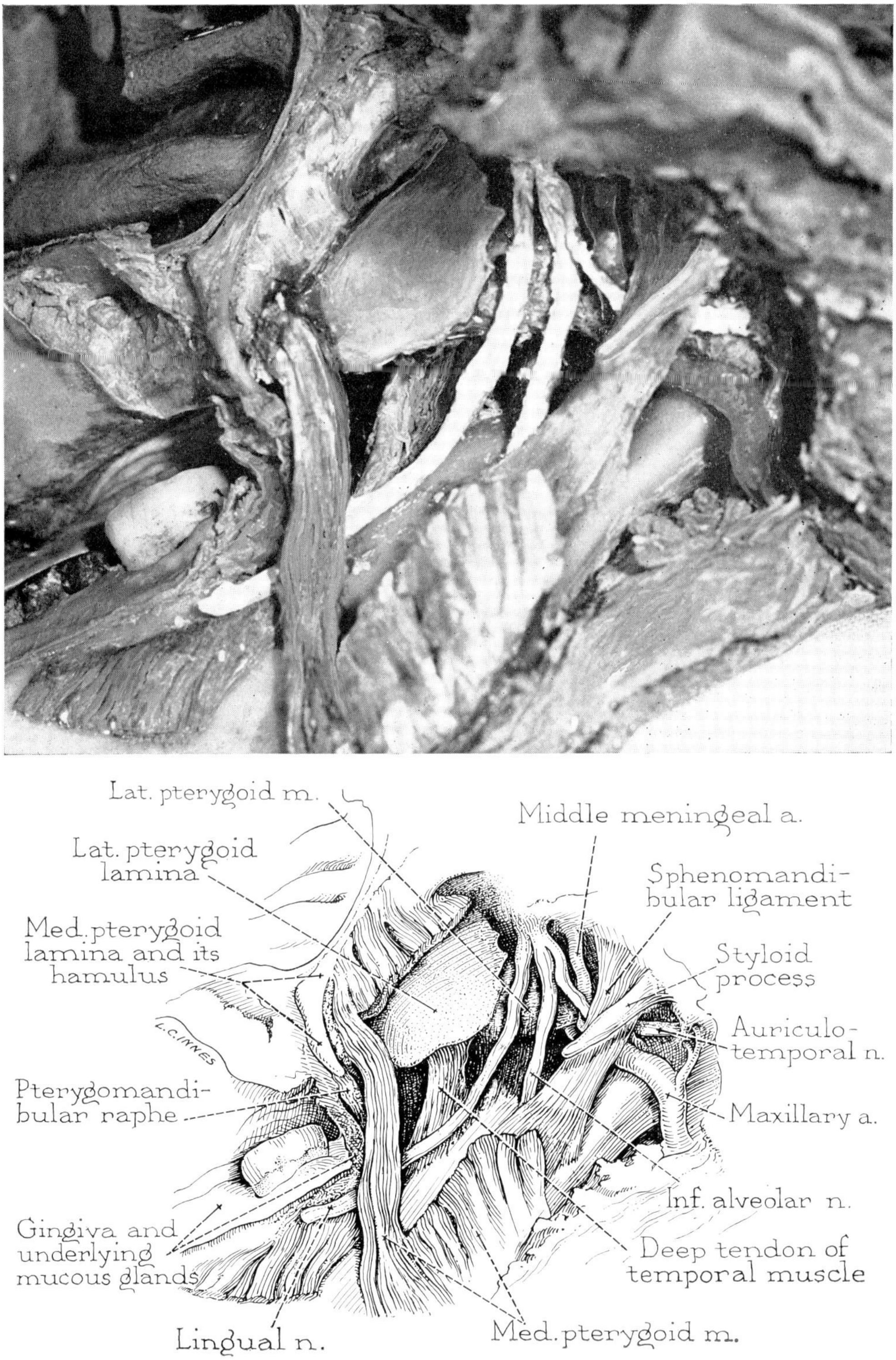

FIG. 4–36. Pterygomandibular space showing deep tendon of temporal muscle.

Continuing anteriorly from the sphenomandibular ligament is a thin fascia which attaches to the lateral lamina of the pterygoid process. The inferior alveolar nerve is attached to the lateral aspect of this interpterygoid fascia (Fig. 4–35). The lingual nerve is attached to the medial side of this fascia. Throughout its length the lingual nerve lies anterior to the inferior alveolar nerve and enters the oral cavity proper through the lingual niche close to the periosteum of the third molar. From the end of the mylohyoid line the pterygomandibular raphe extends to the pterygoid hamulus (Figs. 4–34 and 4–35). The raphe is the junction for the buccinator muscle and the superior constrictor of the pharynx. Covering the thin buccinator muscle just lateral to the raphe is the buccal fat pad which varies greatly in bulk and extent. Along the internal oblique line is attached, like a round firm pole, the deep tendon of the temporalis muscle (Fig. 4–36). The superficial tendon of the temporalis muscle lies along the anterior border of the ramus (Fig. 4–39). The buccal nerve crosses this anterior border about 1 cm above the occlusal plane.

ANESTHESIA FOR MANDIBULAR TISSUES

Inferior Alveolar, Lingual and Buccal Nerve Blocks

Purpose

The blocking of the inferior alveolar nerve is the most important nerve block used in dentistry, simply because there is no other safe method that gives complete anesthesia for the lower posterior teeth. The zone of anesthesia includes the teeth of one half of the mandible, a portion of the buccal gingiva, the skin and mucous membrane of the lower lip, and the skin of the chin. There is often a "fade" so that anesthesia is not complete at the midline. Anesthesia of the lingual gingiva, the adjacent mucosa and the buccal gingiva adjacent to the second premolar and first molar of the lower jaw is usually concomitantly accomplished by the lingual and buccal blocks, respectively.

Technique

Anatomical Approach. MORPHOLOGY. Of all the factors that combine consistently to

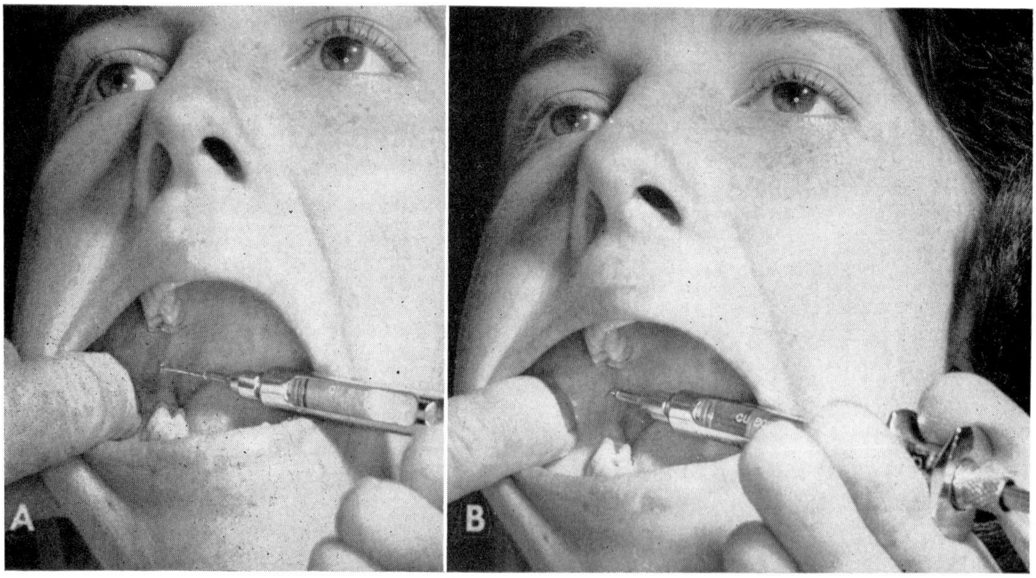

FIG. 4–37. The inferior alveolar nerve block. Note the relaxation of the patient! *A*, Start of injection for the inferior alveolar nerve. *B*, Needle tip at lingula.

produce profound block anesthesia of the inferior alveolar nerve, one is dominant: a working concept of the spatial anatomical relations. The student is advised to study carefully the osteology and the soft structures of the mandible. He should devote particular attention to the course of the inferior alveolar nerve, its branches, and the relationships to both the hard and soft structures.

PREPARATION OF THE PATIENT. The positioning of the patient and the preparation of the tissues for injection are described on page 36.

THE INJECTION. To execute the described anatomical approach successfully, a heavy rigid needle with a short bevel is necessary. The rigid needle acts as a probe and is advocated by such authorities as Sicher,[11] Monheim,[9] and Smith.[13]

The operator's first finger is placed over the fat pad and is used to drag that portion of the pad laterally until the finger comes to rest against the coronoid notch. The area lateral to the raphe is now swabbed with an antiseptic and at the same time palpated for the deep tendon of the temporalis muscle.

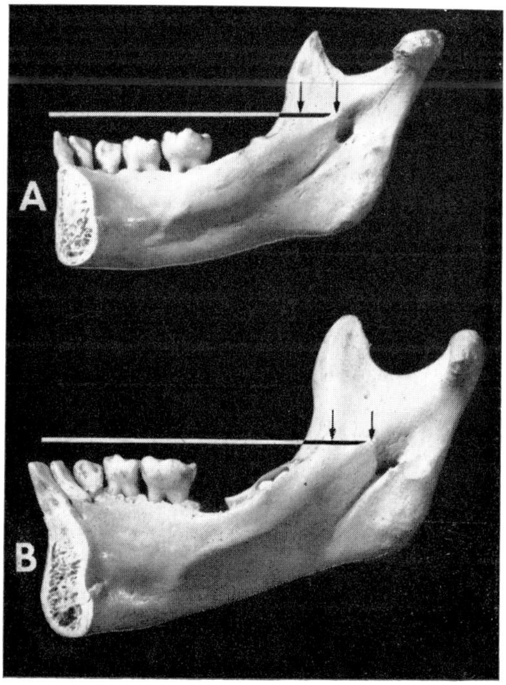

FIG. 4–38. The plane of injection in a child.

Place the syringe over the premolars of the opposite side; puncture the mucosa with the needle at the height indicated by the coronoid notch lateral to the raphe, as near the deep tendon of the temporalis as possible but medial to the fat pad. The moment the needle has penetrated the mucosa, stop, and inject a drop of solution (Fig. 4–38*A*). Wait for 5 seconds and advance the needle slowly about 0.5 cm; gently nudge the needle laterally and feel the deep tendon of the temporalis muscle. From this point to the lingula the distance is 1 cm. Advance the needle a few millimeters further and inject 0.5 ml if it is desired to anesthetize the lingual nerve. Aspiration should be performed. To anesthetize the inferior alveolar nerve, advance the needle and inject a drop or two of the solution before it touches the periosteum anterior to the lingula. After a pause of a few seconds, let the needle slide gently along the periosteum and over the lingular notch into the sulcus and inject 0.5 to 1 ml of the solution (Fig. 4–37*B*). The rate of injection is at least one minute for 1 ml and preferably twice that time. The technique does not vary in the child[16] for the distance from the internal oblique line to the lingula is approximately the same as in the adult (compare Figs. 4–30, 4–33, and 4–38).

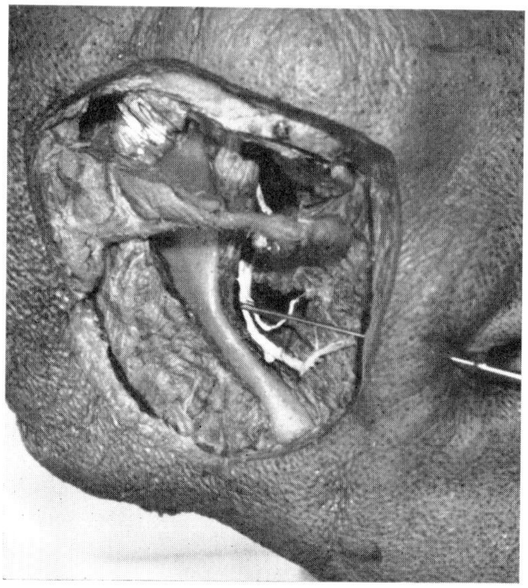

FIG. 4–39. The needle tip at the buccal nerve.

In summary, the direct anatomical approach provides a method of giving an absolutely painless injection during which the patient is not aware of proprioceptive responses. Injury to the lingual nerve is avoided, because the needle passes just medial to the deep tendon. When the needle glides into the sulcus over the lingular notch, it will always be located just lateral to the inferior alveolar nerve, without touching it.[18] The technique has been used by students of Loma Linda University School of Dentistry since 1955 and the evidence for its success is overwhelming.

Direct Thrust Approach. The most commonly used technique for this injection is the so-called direct thrust. It is extremely simple. After having prepared the tissues as previously described, the anesthetist places the tip of his finger or thumb against the coronoid notch and then places the syringe over the contralateral mandibular premolars. Choose the proper height, insert the needle in the mucosa lateral to the raphe, advance it to the floor of the mandibular sulcus, and deposit the solution. Frequently 0.5 ml is reserved to block the lingual nerve as the needle is withdrawn.

Buccal Nerve Block. The buccal nerve may be anesthetized by three different methods:

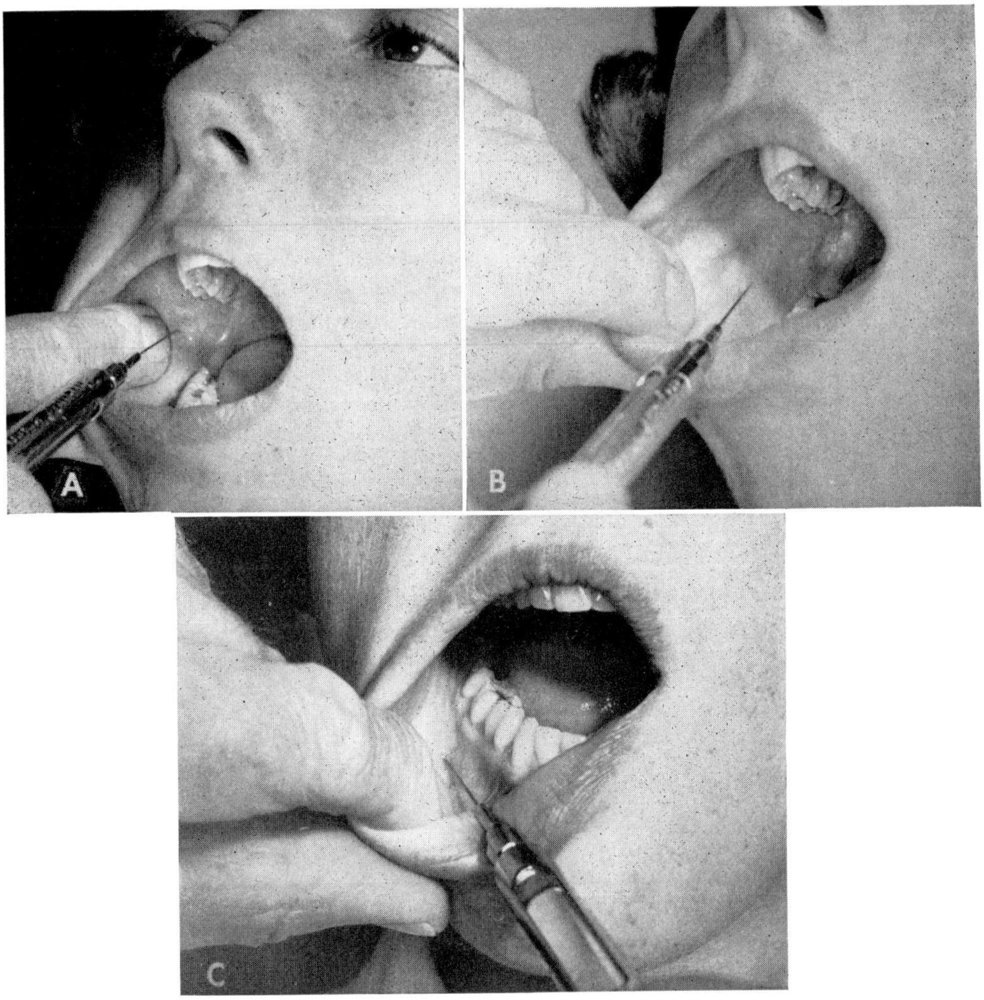

FIG. 4-40. Three techniques for blocking the buccal nerve. *A*, Block just medial to the anterior border of the mandible. *B*, Infiltration 1 cm below the parotid duct. *C*, Infiltration in the vestibule.

(1) The simplest technique is that developed by Sloman.[12] The injection is made about 1 cm above the occlusal plane and a few millimeters medial to the anterior border of the mandible where the buccal nerve passes downward, forward and laterally after it emerges between the two heads of the lateral pterygoid muscle (Figs. 4–39 and 4–40*A*). (2) The injection is submucosal and 1 cm below the parotid duct (Fig. 4–40*B*). The needle is slowly passed distally as the injection is continued. In this manner the terminal branches of the buccal nerve are blocked. Such an approach is necessary when the buccal vestibule or the retromolar area is inflamed or infected, preventing the use of Sloman's technique. (3) The most commonly used method is to make the injection in the buccal vestibule opposite the molars; thus the terminal nerve branches are blocked before they reach the alveolar gingival mucosa (Fig. 4–40*C*).

Cautions

Two major drawbacks to the direct thrust are: (1) The opportunity for injury to the lingual or inferior alveolar nerve is greater than with a direct anatomical approach. (2) The needle penetrates the lower part of the sphenomandibular ligament to enter the sulcus. The entire bevel of the needle may not be lateral to the ligament; therefore the solution may diffuse along the medial aspect of the fascia instead of on the lateral side. Incomplete anesthesia will usually result. Complete anesthesia may occur, the length of time depending upon the rate of diffusion through the sphenomandibular ligament and the interpterygoid fascia. Although the explanation is a theory, it apparently is supported by the research of Berns and Sadove.[2] They reported the course of diffusion of a radiopaque anesthetic solution and with regard to their method concluded: "... It seems that the success of the technique is related to chance."

Always practice aspiration and inject slowly, in minimal volumes.

The Mental and Incisive Nerve Blocks

Purpose

These blocks provide anesthesia for the structures supplied by the terminals of the inferior alveolar nerve when it divides into the incisive and mental nerves at the mental canal. The mental nerve supplies the lip and soft tissue from the first permanent molar to the midline. The incisive nerve supplies the bony structure and the pulps of the premolars, the canine, and the incisors.

Technique

Mental Foramen Block. MORPHOLOGY. The general description of the structures concerned is on page 62. However, a descrip-

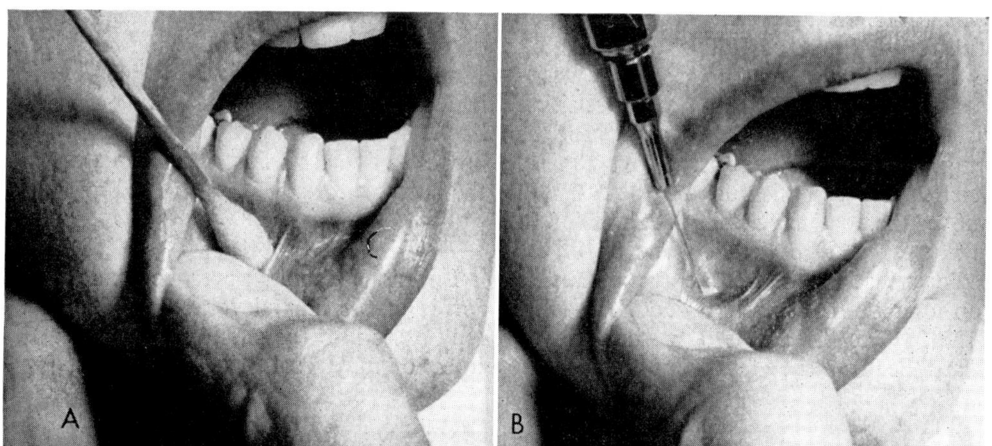

FIG. 4–41. *A*, Cotton-tip applicator used as a probe. *B*, Blocking the mental and incisive nerves at the mental foramen.

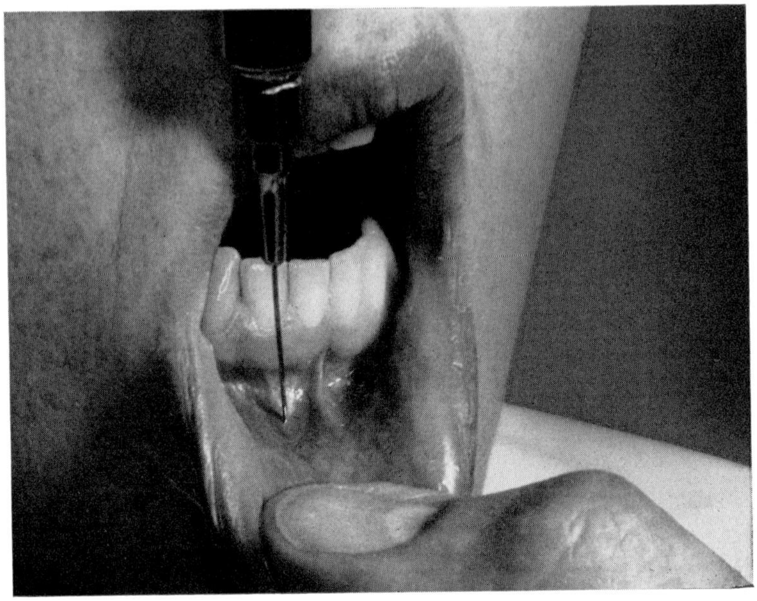

FIG. 4–42. Blocking incisive nerve terminal fibers by diffusion.

tion of the radiographic appearance is of much value, and the student is referred to the description by Worth.[14]

PREPARATION OF THE PATIENT. The positioning of the patient and the preparation of the tissues for injection are described on page 36.

THE INJECTION. The cotton-tip applicator which was used to apply the antiseptic is now used as a probe to find the funnel-like depression into which the mental canal opens. The applicator is held so that it points downward, forward, and medially. After finding the depression the dentist directs the assistant to hold the cotton tip firmly in position (Fig. 4–41*A*). The dentist advances the syringe in the same direction but slightly posterior to the applicator. As the assistant removes the applicator a slight depression of the mucosa will be visible. The tip of the needle is inserted in this depression and a drop or two of solution deposited (Fig. 4–41*B*). The needle is advanced slowly toward the foramen, a few drops are injected, and a few seconds are allowed to elapse before the needle tip slides into the canal. About 0.5 ml is injected slowly into the canal; anesthesia of the teeth anterior to the molars and the facial soft structures will result. The lingual soft structures will sometimes be anesthetized, for which we have no explanation.

Incisive Fossa Block. The efficacy of this injection relates to the small nutrient canals found in the cortical bone in the bottom of the incisive fossa. By depositing the solution in this region *slowly* and not in excess of 1 ml, pulpal and surgical anesthesia of the incisors usually is obtained (Fig. 4–42). If the lingual mucosa requires anesthesia, a small amount of the solution may be injected into the hard mucosa.

Cautions

Injections should never be made at the fornix of the lingual vestibule. The needle may enter into the sublingual gland and an infection may result.

EXTRAORAL NERVE BLOCK

It is our firm conviction that the dentist should be familiar with the extraoral approach to anesthetization of the nerves of the face, jaws, and teeth.

In situations where there are mass casualties it is expected that the dentist exercise his professional training in the anesthetization and care of serious head and face wounds. The extraoral approaches are best from the standpoint of simplicity of technique and of the saving of time. As an example, bilateral infraorbital and mental injections will anesthetize the anterior part of the face. Further, these blocks are much to be preferred to multiple infiltrations in the injured tissue.

The extraoral approach may afford the only means of administering local anesthetic solutions in some situations. The two major situations are (1) trismus and (2) infection. Obviously, the extraoral approach is the easiest if not the only means of effectively rendering anesthesia to large numbers of injured individuals in times of catastrophe. In view of the increasing prevalence of facial traumatic injuries, prudence dictates that every dental student be additionally instructed in the techniques of the extraoral administration of local anesthetics.

Infraorbital Nerve Block

Purpose

Anesthesia provided by this injection covers the area of the distribution of the anterior and middle superior alveolar nerves as well as the terminal cutaneous branches of the nerve. Thus the maxillary teeth and bone anterior to the first permanent molar and the overlying soft tissues of the middle third of the face are affected.

Technique

The morphology has been described on page 49.

The facial tissues should be scrubbed with soap and water followed by alcohol and painted with tincture of Merthiolate. Sterile gloves should be used. A 1-inch sharp thin needle is used for the preliminary injection just lateral to the ala of the nose in the nasolabial sulcus. The index finger is placed to locate the foramen on the right side. The thumb is placed in the nasolabial sulcus and then pressed upward toward the index finger to displace the cheek upward and stretch the skin in preparation for the needle puncture. A short-bevelled 25-gauge 1-inch needle is now advanced through the upward displaced nasolabial sulcus and toward the foramen. A few drops of anesthetic solution are injected at the periphery of the foramen and as the solution wells in the tissue it can be felt by the index finger. Pause 10 seconds until the area is anesthetized, then advance the needle 1 or 2 mm into the canal. Over a period of two minutes inject 0.5 to 1 ml while the finger is pressed over the foramen so that the solution must diffuse posteriorly along the neurovascular bundle. The described maneuvers remove the facial vein from the path of the needle and allow the needle to follow the plane of least resistance as it advances between the levator labii superioris and levator anguli oris muscles (Fig. 4–17). On the left side, the anesthetist approaches from behind the patient's head, his thumb locates the foramen, and his index finger is placed in the nasolabial sulcus.

Maxillary Nerve Block

Purpose

The purpose of this block has been described in connection with the intraoral approach on page 58.

Technique

The preliminary procedures of preparation are the same as for the infraorbital nerve block. The points of entry suggested by Braun[3] and Smith[13] seem simplest. Draw a 2-cm horizontal line parallel with the lower border of the zygomatic bone. Intersect it with the upper end of a 2-cm line drawn parallel to the anterior surface of the mandibular coronoid process. Connect the horizontal and vertical lines to form a triangle. The central point within the triangle is the puncture point for the entrance of the 6-cm 20-gauge short-bevelled needle fitted with a rubber stop or marker near the hub. According to Sicher[11] the needle point is advanced along the tuberosity until it is stopped by the lateral pterygoid plate (Fig. 4–43*A*). The rubber stopper or marker is

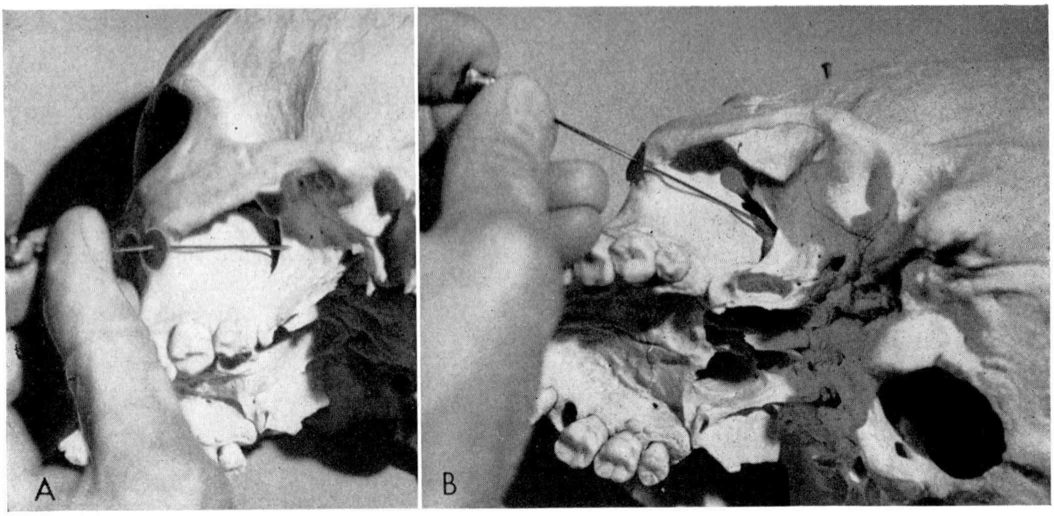

FIG. 4–43. *A*, Measuring the distance to the lateral pterygoid plate. *B*, Needle directed to fossa.

now placed 5 mm from the skin. The needle then is slightly withdrawn, and directed anteriorly and slightly superiorly and advanced through the pterygopalatine fissure 5 mm into the pterygopalatine fossa (Fig. 4–43*B*). Two to 4 ml of anesthetic solution are usually sufficient, depending on the agent used and the proximity to the nerve. The technique of Sicher[11] prevents advancing the needle through the sphenopalatine foramen into the nasal cavity. Obviously, such a penetration could result in contamination of the pterygopalatine fossa with resultant infection.

If the injection is made as the needle approaches the tuberosity, then the area of effect may be limited to the field of innervation of the posterior superior alveolar nerve.

Inferior Alveolar Nerve Block

The points of reference are marked extraorally to determine the direction and depth of needle insertion. The coronoid notch is palpated with one finger or the thumb placed intraorally. The anterior border of the ramus and coronoid notch is then determined by palpation, employing the opposed first finger and thumb. The skin is marked with a surgical pencil to designate the spot from which a horizontal line is drawn to the posterior border of the mandibular ramus, parallel with the inferior border of the mandible. A cross is marked slightly posterior to the middle of this horizontal line. The mark designates the middle of the mandibular sulcus, in line with the lingula. From the "midpoint mark" a line is drawn parallel to the posterior border of the ramus and extending to a point below the inferior border of the mandible. The inferior point must allow the needle to pass superiorly and on the medial side of the body and ramus of the mandible. The distance between the point of puncture and the horizontal line first established is now measured. A sterile marker on the needle is adjusted for that distance. It is presumed that the patient has received premedication. The soft tissue at the puncture point is anesthetized with a preliminary injection. For the deep injection a heavy, rigid 22- or 23-gauge, 3-inch needle is directed immediately upward to the area of the sulcus, previously marked on the horizontal line. After the needle is in the proper position the Luer syringe is attached and 1 to 2 ml of solution injected. Every attempt is made to avoid injecting into the muscle fibers in order to avoid post-injection trismus.

Mental Nerve Block

The tissues are prepared as before described. The point of insertion of the needle

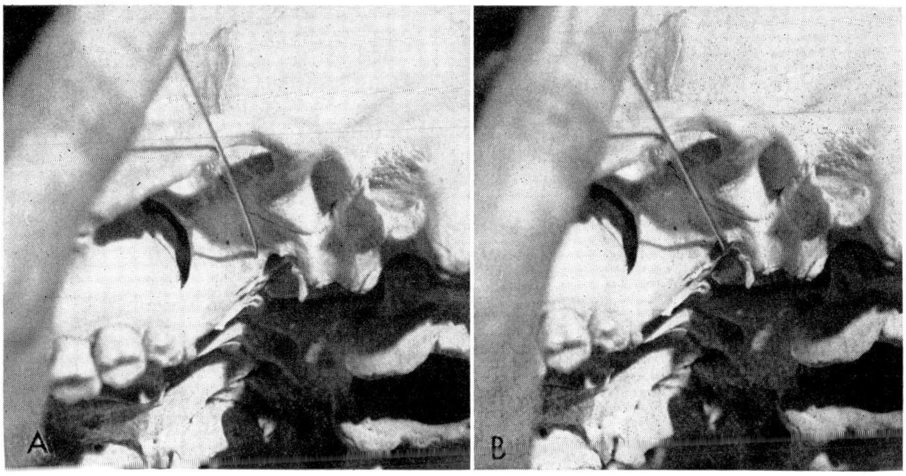

FIG. 4–44. The extraoral mandibular nerve block. *A*, Needle tip at lateral pterygoid plate. *B*, Needle tip at foramen ovale.

is just distal to the second mandibular premolar. The needle points anteriorly, medially, and inferiorly. The needle is moved toward the foramen, injection being made slowly ahead of the point. The point of contact with the periosteum will be slightly above the midpoint as measured from the gingival margin of the teeth to the inferior border of the mandible. From the apical portion of the second premolar the needle slides forward and downward into the foramen. It must be remembered that fibers from the cervical plexus provide some innervation in the submental area of the chin. Supplementary anesthesia will be required if the submental area is involved.

Mandibular Nerve Block

Following a preliminary injection a heavy (20-gauge), long (60-mm) needle is inserted in the center of the half-circle formed by the lower border of the zygomatic arch and the sharp upper border of the mandibular ramus (mandibular notch). Smith[13] stresses that the needle must be held at right angles to the surface of the skin as it is advanced. The needle will meet the mandibular nerve about 1 cm anterior to the foramen ovale (Fig. 4–44).

BIBLIOGRAPHY

1. *Accepted Dental Therapeutics*, 33rd ed. Chicago, American Dental Association, 1969/70, pp. 42–43.
2. Berns, J. M. and Sadove, M. S.: Mandibular block injection: a method of study using an injected radiopaque material. J. Amer. Dent. Assoc. *65*:735, 1962.
3. Braun, Heinrich and Harris, M. L. (translator): *Local Anesthesia*, 2nd English ed. Philadelphia, Lea & Febiger, 1924.
4. Fischer, Guido and Riethmuller, R. H.: *Local Anesthesia in Dentistry*. Philadelphia, Lea & Febiger, 1923.
5. Hayden, Jess, Jr.: The innervation of the maxillary first permanent and primary molars as determined by the deposition of local anesthetic solutions. Acta Odont. Scand. *23*:147, 1965.
6. Jorgensen, N. B.: Measurements for intraoral block of the maxillary nerve. J. Oral Surg. *6*:1, 1948.
7. Jorgensen, N. B.: Accidental intravenous injection of procaine in dentistry. J. Southern Calif. Dent. Assoc. *20*:17, 1952.
8. Jorgensen, N. B. and Hughes, J. E.: Measurements of the ramus of the mandible in relation to the inferior alveolar block. J. Oral Surg. *10*:318, 1952.
9. Monheim, L. M.: *Local Anesthesia and Pain Control in Dental Practice*, 2nd ed. St. Louis, C. V. Mosby Co., 1961.
10. Nevin, Mendel and Burgoyne, J. R.: *Conduction, Infiltration and General Anesthesia in Dentistry*, 6th ed. Brooklyn, Dental Items of Interest, 1959, p. 230.
11. Sicher, Harry and Dubrul, E. L.: *Oral*

Anatomy, 5th ed. St. Louis, C. V. Mosby Co., 1970.

12. Sloman, E. G.: Anatomy and anesthesia of the buccinator (long buccal) nerve. J. Amer. Dent. Assoc. *26*:428, 1939.
13. Smith, A. E.: *Block Anesthesia and Allied Subjects.* St. Louis, C. V. Mosby Co., c1920, p. 527.
14. Worth, H. M.: *Principles and Practice of Oral Radiologic Interpretation.* Chicago, Year Book Medical Publishers, Inc., 1963, p. 67.

Films

15. Jorgensen, N. B. and Hughes, John: Local anesthesia in dentistry (maxillary considerations). 16 mm, sound, color, 30 min. Chicago, Amer. Dent. Assoc. Film Libr. 1953.
16. Jorgensen, N. B., Hayden, Jess, Jr., and Roberts, W. H.: Local anesthesia in dentistry for children. 16 mm, sound, color, 22 min. Chicago, Amer. Dent. Assoc. Film Libr. 1959.
17. Jorgensen, N. B., Burns, A. E., Roberts, W. H., and Mitchell, R. P.: Maxillary nerve block. 16 mm, color, sound, 18 min. Chicago, Amer. Dent. Assoc. Film. Libr. 1963.
18. Jorgensen, N. B., Mitchell, R. P, Hughes, John, and Roberts, W. H.: Inferior alveolar, lingual and buccal nerve blocks. 16 mm, color, sound, 22 min. Chicago, Amer. Dent. Assoc. Film Libr. 1964.

Chapter

5

Complications from Sedation and Local Anesthesia*

LOCAL COMPLICATIONS
- **Contamination of Needles**
- **Reactions to Topical or Injected Solutions**
- **Breakage of Needles**
- **Lip-Chewing**
- **Emphysema**
- **Trauma of Injection**
- **Bleeding Due to Hemophilia or Anticoagulant Therapy**

SYSTEMIC COMPLICATIONS
- **Allergic Reactions**
- **Toxic Reactions**
- **Psychic Reactions**
- **Serum Hepatitis**

DISCUSSION
- **Inferior Alveolar Nerve Block**
- **Posterior Superior Alveolar Nerve Block**
- **Maxillary Nerve Block**
- **Hypertension, Cardiovascular or Cerebral Disease**
- **Inhalation and Intravenous Sedation**

PROPHYLAXIS AND TREATMENT
- **Management of Toxic Reactions**

SUMMARY AND CONCLUSIONS

The purpose of this chapter is to set forth in a classified form and to discuss the complications which may accompany or follow the injection of solutions used for sedation or as local anesthetics. The classification and the discussion relate to our observations made in the course of the clinical practice of dentistry.

The use of local anesthetics in dentistry has become such a routine procedure in the average office that one is apt to ignore possible hazards in its employment. Although it does appear to be without any dangers, complications do occasionally occur. These complications may be classified as: (1) local and (2) systemic.

A more extensive bibliography is readily available in Accepted Dental Therapeutics[1] which is conveniently divided into sections concerning: (1) the general principles of medication, including emergency treatment and sterilization; (2) therapeutic agents; (3) therapeutic aids; (4) therapeutic guides; and (5) section indexes.

LOCAL COMPLICATIONS

Contamination of Needles

Bacterial contamination of needles is a relatively infrequent occurrence in meticulous dental operatories since the introduction of disposable needles. Its usual sequela is a *low-grade infection*, whether confined to the area of the attached periodontal tissues or deeply situated in the intratemporal space. Improper techniques or methods of handling by the assistant or dentist lead to varying degrees of contamination. If the needle is contaminated while outside the mouth, or through repeated deep injections, severe infections can result. Contamination of needles used in intravenous injection may result in abscess or slough.

* Footnote on page 89.

Chemical deposits on the needle are due to sterilizing solutions, or perhaps chemical vapor sterilization. Inflammation and pain are frequent after-effects.

Reactions to Topical or Injected Solutions

Local reactions to topical or injected solutions are usually seen as *epithelial desquamation* following the application of topical anesthetics. Such desquamation usually results from too long an application of the topical anesthetic, but may be due to a heightened sensitivity of the tissue. All local anesthetics are toxic. The after-effects are usually transitory. *Sterile abscesses* or gangrene may develop owing to ischemia resulting from injecting an excess of anesthetic solution with its contained vasoconstrictor into the firm, hard tissue of the palate (Fig. 5–1*A*). *Local allergic reactions* such as blisters on the oral mucosa or lips are to be considered as warning signs; further use of the causative agents should be accompanied with suitable precautions, and a change to a local anesthetic of different chemical structure. *Dentists are not immune to contact dermatitis. Trismus and pain* follow the injection of solutions into muscles and tendons, and they are among the variety of local tissue changes produced by the local anesthetics. Much of the frequent soreness attributed to postsurgical operative causes is simply the result of improper administration of solutions. A further complication, similarly related to failure to adhere to principles of injection based on morphology, is post-injection *paresthesia* and/or *neuritis* caused by the needle penetrating or scratching the nerve. These same untoward effects may occur during intravenous sedation, particularly in the antecubital fossae.

Breakage of Needles

Breakage of needles is seldom a problem. Needles available today possess the physical qualities to prevent such a mishap. Breakage which does occur is usually the result of the impaling of muscular tissue or of passing beneath the periosteum; such mishaps cause a sudden reflex movement of the patient's head, during which the needle is snapped off. Reason dictates the use of long hubs for long needles used with cartridge syringes.

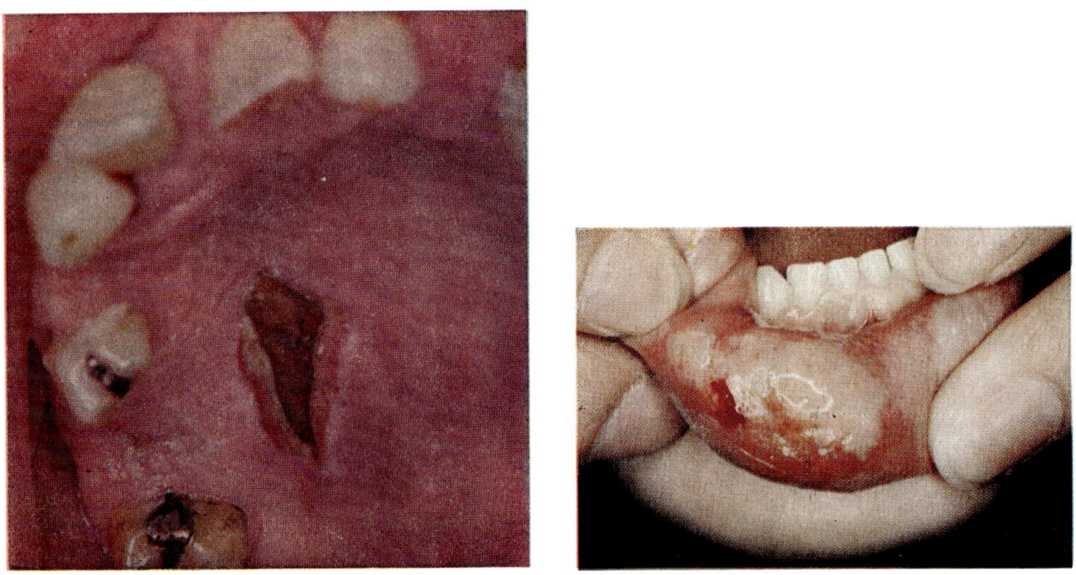

FIG. 5–1. *A*, Ulcer at injection site. (Schaffer, Julius, Calman, H. I., and Levy, Bernard: Dent. Radiog. Photog. *39*:9, 1966.) *B*, Lip-biting following inferior alveolar injection, child aged 7. (Courtesy Assoc. Prof. R. Johnson, D.D.S. Dept. of Pedodontics, Univ. of Iowa.)

Lip-Chewing

Lip-chewing is a complication occurring in children (Fig. 5–1*B*). It is due to the use of the long-acting local anesthetics employed for these patients. The after-effects can be most unpleasant for the child, his parents, and the dentist. Many dentists routinely employ long-acting anesthetics in order to obtain profundity of effect. The child should always be sedated prior to the injection if dismissal from the dental office long precedes the dissipation of the anesthetic action. For brief appointments the use of short-acting solutions should be routine. Even so, a cotton roll should be placed between the lips or tied to the vestibule by means of dental floss or sutures passed through the dental embrasures if anesthesia exists at the time of dismissal. Verbal warnings to the child or accompanying adult should be explicitly expressed, but may be futile if not reinforced by use of the cotton roll.

Emphysema

Emphysema uncommonly occurs after an injection.[18] An example is that of a 10-year-old boy who received an inferior alveolar injection. Within two hours of his dismissal, the child returned to the office exhibiting homolateral swelling and crepitation in the anterior triangle of the neck and the face. The dentist and the consulting pediatrician shared mutually the amazement at this sequela of dental treatment, and prescribed antihistaminics on the basis of a possible allergic response. Questioning revealed that the boy had been blowing up balloons immediately after his dental treatment. The manner in which the symptoms subsided suggested that air in the fascial planes, rather than allergy, was the cause.

Trauma of Injection

The trauma of injection comprises the vast majority of local complications. Reactions from the supraperiosteal technique are generally minor, consisting of edema and after-pain and sometimes slight ulceration at the puncture point. The former is due to infection, too rapid an injection, or too large a volume; the latter is due to an infection. The unpleasantness generally passes in a few days. Hematomas may result from nicking an artery. Usually the effects are seen in connection with the posterior superior alveolar artery and less commonly the facial. Obviously, any of these local complications can result in swelling and pain. Two common techniques of administration often cause pain, the first because of lack of skill of administration; the second is irrevocably tied to morphology and physiology: The complications from the palatine injections are mostly immediate pain from the needle insertion; subperiosteal injections may result in lifting the periosteum from the bone, causing after-pain and even infection. From a physiological standpoint, this injection is contraindicated.

The use of sharp, thin, disposable needles predisposes to hematomas and trismus, for arteries and muscles or tendons are easily penetrated with these much too flexible instruments. The use of such needles, coupled with an improper technique, may result in a retromandibular injection in the parotid region (see Fig. 8–5*a*, page 116). Among the most usual sequelae are transitory paralysis of branches of the facial nerve or a mild parotitis. More serious complications may include neuritis or long-lasting nerve paralysis and a severe parotitis.

Extravascular injections of drugs used for sedation may be quite irritating. *Hematomas* occur, particularly with the sharp, long-bevelled needles used for intravenous injection. They may be accompanied by some discomfort, but usually are harmless, with an unsightly discoloration being evident. *Thrombosis* and *thrombophlebitis* may occur as a result of bacterial contamination or irritation to the intima of the vein due to very large needles, improper positioning of needles, irritating solutions or too-rapid injection. Finally, *arterial injection* is the greatest hazard and even a few minims of solution will almost immediately cause a burning pain distally in the hand and fingers with blanching of the skin. (This should not be confused with the mild tingling or irritation which occasionally is experienced as the solutions pass centrally in the venous channel.) If the spasm continues and is left untreated, the eventual result may be gangrene.

Bleeding Due to Hemophilia or Anticoagulant Therapy

Bleeding due to hemophilia or anticoagulant therapy is always a hazard. The first is readily recognized by both the patient and the dentist. The latter is much more prevalent, but is not so well recognized. It is particularly a danger when deep block injections are required for the relief of pain in an active ambulatory patient. These patients should not receive any deep injections or intravenous sedation in the dental office.

SYSTEMIC COMPLICATIONS

Allergic Reactions

Allergic reactions are extremely uncommon. *Anaphylaxis* presents the gravest challenge, for the opportunity to render support to the patient is so fleeting that death usually results. Fortunately, anaphylactic shock is known by its rarity with regard to anesthetic solutions. *Skin eruptions* may occasionally be a manifestation of allergy.

Toxic Reactions

Toxic reactions appear systemically if too large an amount of an anesthetic drug is absorbed too rapidly into the system. Absorption is increased when too much solution is injected too rapidly into the highly vascular circumoral tissues. Further, it is accepted that the intravenous injection of local anesthetics increases the probability of a toxic reaction.[1] As Harris reported, many dentists, because of the small volumes they inject, believe that: (1) there will be no toxic reactions, and (2) the advantages of rapid injection outweigh the disadvantages. The error of such thinking lies in the demonstrable evidence that ordinarily a dental anesthetic injected intravenously "... is 15 times in excess of the maximal safe rate, or over 200 times more toxic."[8] Procaine, an ester, has now largely been replaced by local anesthetics containing an amide linkage (see Chap. 9). Used in the same concentration as procaine, amides are more toxic. Further, a reaction may occur either to the intravenously injected local anesthetic or to the vasoconstrictor, or to both. Adriani and Campbell[2] reported that the effect of spray or paste topical anesthetics may simulate the effect of intravenous injection. Further, these sprays come in high concentrations, up to 10 per cent, which in itself enormously increases the toxicity. Spray products apparently are no more effective in producing anesthesia than those applied with a swab; but sprays do have several disadvantages which may introduce unnecessary hazard in their use.[1] In any case, the toxic reaction sequence may take the form of stimulation, convulsions, and depression.

Intravenous injections of atropine and scopolamine are apt to damage glaucomatous eyes.[7,13] Toxic doses of these drugs promptly produce effects. Those seen in the dental office usually include a dry and burning mouth, marked thirst, and a skin that is flushed, hot and dry. A rash may develop, especially noticeable on the head and neck. Restlessness and hallucinations may occur. Strangely enough, scopolamine, which is considered a sedative, may in ordinary therapeutic doses produce these effects, probably due to idiosyncrasy.[7] In summary, from the standpoint of dental practice, the patient who experiences these reactions may be described as "red as a beet, dry as a bone and wild as a hare." Fortunately, these drugs have a wide margin of safety and such reactions are extremely rare in our experience.

Meperidine is often administered in 50-mg dosages and in this amount, if rapidly injected intravenously, may cause severe untoward reactions including dizziness, restlessness, flushing and tremors, respiratory depression, nausea, vomiting and even convulsions and syncope. With slowly administered analgesic doses, the patient may experience minor transitory effects such as flushing of the face and drying of the mouth. Its interaction with other drugs is clinically significant. When injected with phenothiazines there may be an exaggeration of the respiratory depressant effect, and during intravenous sedation its effect is enhanced by the previously administered barbiturate. There is a serious potentiation of its narcotic effect by monoamine oxidase inhibitors.[13]

Pentobarbital sodium injected intravenously can cause respiratory depression. More often the observed effect of a heavy dose is a prolonged drowsiness, which is often described as a "hangover" in contradistinction to the pleasant and short-acting drowsiness associated with sedation. Hyperalgesia may be observed if sedative doses are not supplemented by local anesthesia.

Interactions of various drugs often produce adverse reactions. A current and classic example is the interaction of meperidine and the monoamine oxidase inhibitors (MAOI). The MAOI drugs potentiate the action of sedatives, hypnotics, tranquilizers, narcotics and pressor amines. Conversely, many of the phenothiazines antagonize narcotic-induced analgesia; for instance, promethazine (Phenergan) and prochlorperazine (Compazine) exhibit marked to slight antianalgesia, respectively.[13] The complications from the inhalation of nitrous oxide and oxygen are related to hypoxia, or the bringing of the patient into the excitement (Guedel's second stage) state of anesthesia or deeper. Rarely, nitric oxide will be found in cylinders of N_2O. The impurity produces methemoglobinemia and pulmonary edema. Although it is stated that this danger is virtually eliminated in the United States, from abroad there have been reports of death attributed to nitric oxide.[6]

Psychic Reactions

Psychic reactions are exhibited by most patients, but dentists usually notice only those signs which immediately precede *syncope*. Fortunately, first-aid procedures for syncope are so ingrained into most people and the recuperative powers of the body are such that shock seldom ensues. Syncope can lead to *secondary shock*. The latter, if not treated immediately, can pass to an irreversible state, all within the confines of the dental office.

Acute asthmatic attacks may follow the administration of a local anesthetic. Such attacks are considered to be due to allergy or emotional stress.

Serum Hepatitis

The incidence of serum hepatitis is increasing rapidly. The disease is transmitted solely by parenteral introduction of the virus, and there have been reports of many well-documented cases following the use of nonsterile injection needles and syringes.[1]

DISCUSSION

To better illustrate what may happen during the deep injection of a local anesthetic solution, the path of the needle during three injections is described.

Inferior Alveolar Nerve Block

When administering the inferior alveolar injection, the mucous membrane at the area of the needle insertion should be wiped clean with sterile gauze and an antiseptic applied, such as tincture of Merthiolate. If saliva flows copiously at the time of needle insertion, bacteria may be introduced into the deeper structures, and though these may be relatively harmless to the host, a low-grade infection and after-pain may be the result. To minimize this invasion, a roll of sterile gauze should be placed in the upper vestibule blocking the parotid duct, and a second pad of gauze underneath the tongue over the salivary caruncle. Bacteria of a more harmful nature may be also introduced by the inadvertent touch of the needle point to any foreign object such as a finger or lips, or by the repeated use of the same needle for deep injections. The bacteria, once introduced into the infratemporal space, may cause an infection both serious and difficult to treat.

1. The path of the needle is through loose areolar tissue. If the needle is inserted or directed too far medially, it will enter the medial pterygoid muscle (Fig. 8–5*B*), resulting in trismus, after-pain

and probably incomplete anesthesia or none at all.

2. If the needle is directed too far laterally, it will penetrate the deep tendon of the temporalis muscle (Fig. 4–36). Trismus and after-pain may be expected. Furthermore, if the needle is continued in this too-lateral path, it will be rammed against the periosteum, and the result will be pain and a reflex action by the patient which may result in needle breakage.
3. If the needle is directed in a path diverging inferiorly from a plane through the coronoid notch, the deepest point of the concavity of the anterior border of the ramus (Fig. 4–33), it will have to penetrate the sphenomandibular ligament, which covers the mandibular sulcus (Figs. 4–34 and 4–35). If the entire bevel of the needle is not lateral to the sphenomandibular ligament, solution is deposited along its medial aspect, and incomplete anesthesia of the inferior alveolar nerve is the result although anesthesia for the lingual nerve may be profound.

The inferior alveolar nerve or the lingual nerve may be traumatized by the needle. These nerves, if accidentally rammed by the needle, do not slide away, as is generally supposed, since they are both attached firmly to the interpterygoid fascia, a structure which continues forward from the anterior border of the sphenomandibular ligament to the lateral pterygoid lamina. When the mouth is kept wide open, the interpterygoid fascia is stretched and holds the two nerves quite firmly, as if on a trellis (see Fig. 4–35).

To avoid injury to the lingual nerve the needle must be inserted at the proper level, relative to the coronoid notch, kept close to the medial aspect of the deep tendon of the temporalis muscle and lateral to the pterygomandibular raphe.

To avoid injury to the inferior alveolar nerve a heavy, rigid needle with a short bevel should touch the periosteum just before reaching the lingular notch and then slide gently over this saddle-like bony surface into the anterior part of the sulcus (Fig. 4–33). If the needle is advanced posteriorly into the mandibular sulcus, the inferior alveolar artery or vein may be punctured and injected into. The result may be a local hematoma or a systemic toxic reaction from the injected drug. If the lingual and inferior alveolar nerves are injured, paresthesia or postanesthetic neuritis may result. These complications can be avoided by confining the needle tip to the anterior part of the sulcus. Injection into the vessel must be avoided by aspirating before injecting.[10,15]

Posterior Superior Alveolar Nerve Block

The posterior superior alveolar nerve block is a simple and effective injection that recently has been abandoned by many dentists because of the increased frequency of hematomas. These are due to the 27- or 30-gauge, pointed, long-bevelled needles which are now in vogue and demand, and which make it impossible to detect and follow anatomical landmarks. For instance, from just distal of the zygomatic process the point of the needle must be advanced medially, superiorly, and posteriorly along the periosteum toward the foramina located halfway between the upper and lower border of the maxilla (Fig. 4–20*B*). Here the tuberosity makes a sharp turn medially and, if the needle advances further, the pterygoid venous plexus or the maxillary artery may be punctured (Fig. 4–23). If the syringe and needle are kept in a plane parallel with the sagittal plane, the maxillary artery and/or the lateral pterygoid muscle may be invaded by the needle. Obviously, trismus and hematoma are possible complications of this injection if the needle deviates from the proper path, and it will with a 27- or 30-gauge $1\frac{3}{8}''$ needle. Only with a heavy rigid needle with a short bevel can the proper anatomical path routinely be followed, as with a probe.

Maxillary Nerve Block

When the maxillary nerve block is executed through the greater palatine canal (Figs. 4–27 and 4–28), care must be exercised that the needle does not penetrate the thin lateral wall of the nasal cavity. Not only will there be no anesthesia, but infection may also be the result. When directed laterally, the needle and solution may enter the infratemporal space and the pterygoid muscle through the pterygomaxillary fissure. Trismus will result. If the needle is in the correct path but advanced too far, the orbital cavity may be entered. Solution injected here may temporarily paralyze the muscles of the eyeball; even the optic nerve may be anesthetized, resulting in temporary blindness. If obstructions in the canal are encountered when giving this injection, the needle should not be forced or needle breakage may result. The alternative path is along the tuberosity. The most common complication will be severe hematoma if the maxillary artery is punctured. Also, the orbit might be entered if the needle is advanced too far. These complications can be avoided by Smith's[16] and Jorgensen's[9] technique and determination of the depth of needle insertion.

A most serious complication is postinjection infection; asepsis must be most carefully maintained when using this injection.

Hypertension, Cardiovascular or Cerebral Disease

The treatment of patients with hypertension, cardiovascular or cerebral disease is increasingly common. Hypertensives are a problem because they exhibit a great lability of blood pressure. The anticipation of dental treatment causes an initial elevation of the blood pressure which may be heightened by the stimulus of an injection or dental treatment. However, the underlying cause is endogenous epinephrine.

Patients with a history of *cardiovascular* or *cerebrovascular disease* suffer an elevation in blood pressure after any noxious stimulus, Obviously, any rise in blood pressure may be dangerous for these patients. The reports of Cheraskin and Prasertsuntarasai,[5] McCarthy,[11] and our observations of dental clinic patients at Loma Linda University since 1955 confirm the fact that the blood pressure is not elevated by the small amount of vasoconstrictor (1:100,000 to 1:50,000) contained in the most commonly employed dental anesthetic solutions.

Warnings against the use of vasoconstrictors such as epinephrine are still heard. Many of these are repetitions based on early teachings such as those expressed by Berlove.[3] More recently the question frequently has been asked if patients taking monoamino oxidase inhibitors (see Chap. 3) can tolerate the epinephrine in a local anesthetic solution. It is reported that "there is no danger in giving a reasonable amount of local anesthetic containing vasoconstrictor."[17]

Inhalation and Intravenous Sedation

The techniques of intravenous and inhalation sedation are often misunderstood and frequently abused. The main purpose of these techniques is to eliminate anxiety and fear of dentistry. When pain is anticipated, local anesthesia should be used to control the pain. Only if the dentist is trained in general anesthesia should nitrous oxide and oxygen sedation (analgesia) be supplemented with sedatives or narcotics, for the patient may readily slip into general anesthesia. Because of the increasing awareness of the interaction of drugs, the dentist should keep current through such texts as Modell's *Drugs of Choice*,[13] *The Medical Letter on Drugs and Therapeutics*[12] (in Britain *The Drug and Therapeutic Bulletin*) and the informative *Physician's Desk Reference* (PDR),[14] which, of course, is not a critical guide.

PROPHYLAXIS AND TREATMENT

Prophylaxis and treatment of many of the local complications have been altered by the introduction of disposable needles. For instance, bacterial contamination could be completely eliminated if dental assistants properly handled solutions, needles and syringes and the dentist exercised meticulous care during injections. At the same time, however, long-bevelled needles with a sharp-pointed end do increase the hazard of inadvertently entering tissues that should be avoided (Fig. 5–2) whether the injection is for the purpose of local anesthesia or intravenous sedation. In either case the proper needle should be chosen (see pages 38 and 32). By choosing veins in the dorsum of the hand, the cephalic vein in the forearm or the median cephalic vein at the antecubital fossa, the risk of intra-arterial injection is avoided. The aspiration of blood should always precede injection. Each dentist should select some means of stabilizing the arm or hand which is to receive the injection. If an intra-arterial injection should accidentally occur, great care must be taken to stabilize the painfully affected arm while leaving the needle in the artery in order to inject up to 10 ml of 1 per cent procaine solution to break the spasm. If this does not ease the pain and relax the spasm permanently, the patient must be referred to a competent physician for possible hospitalization and treatment. Obviously a record of the time, the anatomical site and the dose and concentration of the solution must be kept and a copy furnished to the attending physician.

The passage for the needle in giving deep injections, such as the inferior alveolar, tuberosity, or infraorbital injections, is through loose, fatty, areolar tissue. In our hands, thin needles with long, pointed bevels cannot be used as probes during the injection of local anesthetics and may easily invade a muscle, artery, or nerve. Trismus and after-pain, hematoma, paresthesia, or postanesthetic neuritis may follow.

The problem of *needle breakage* is rare, but

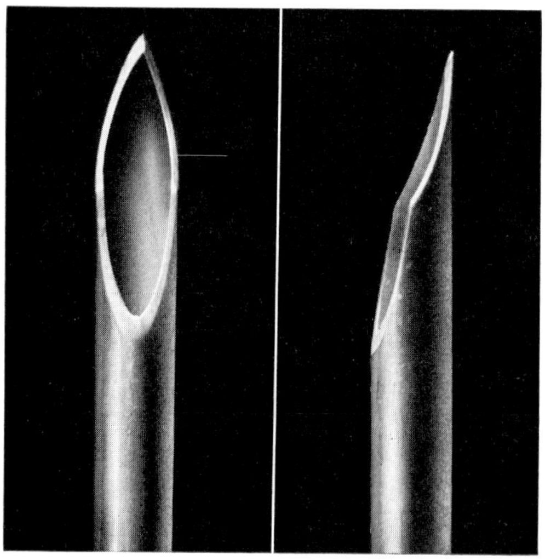

FIG. 5–2. Long-bevelled needle.

if it occurs the protruding needle should be grasped with a needle forceps before it disappears in the tissue. Such forceps should always be at hand. If the needle end is not protruding, the jaw should be immobilized and the consultation of an oral surgeon immediately sought.

The *prophylaxis for trismus* consists in adhering strictly to the correct anatomical route for the needle, which is impossible without the use of a heavy rigid needle with a short bevel, preferably a Mizzy* conical or a 23-gauge disposable Huber point, short-bevelled needle, manufactured by Cook-Waite (Fig. 4–2). The *proper treatment for trismus and neuritis*, in our experience, is infrared radiation. The paresthesia which may follow the injury to the nerve will pass in a few weeks. We are convinced that when injecting local anesthetics *hematomas* can largely be avoided by the use of a heavy, rigid needle with a short bevel. Such a needle will transmit a sensation if it touches the resistant wall of the artery. If this is noted the needle can then be slightly withdrawn and a new path taken. A vein may be penetrated but this does not result in hematoma. However, aspiration must be done to avoid systemic reactions.[1,10] If the technique is carelessly executed, infection may result. This infection can be serious and at times difficult to control. Mizzy conical needles were used by dental students in the Oral Surgery Department of Loma Linda University for approximately ten years, during which time only one hematoma was observed. When disposable needles became mandatory for student use, 7 cases of hematoma occurred during the first trial period of 500 injections in the surgery clinic. The disposable needles were 23-gauge with long, pointed bevels. *The treatment of hematoma* in the region of the maxillary tuberosity starts with control of the bleeding by placing gauze, packed under pressure, in the buccal vestibule, and applying extraoral pressure over the swollen area. Later treatment includes the use of infrared rays; possible benefits are obtained from the local injection

* Mizzy Corporation, Clifton Forge, Va. and Cook-Waite Laboratories, Inc., New York, N.Y, 10016.

of hyaluronidase after the swelling has stabilized, and it has been ascertained that there is no infection.

Prevention is the best *treatment for hematomas following intravenous injection.* Other methods are to apply and maintain pressure with a Band-Aid as soon as the needle is withdrawn. In case of an *extravascular injection*, there may be considerable stinging pain which can be relieved by the injection of 1 to 3 ml of a 1 per cent procaine solution. In case of *thrombus* and mild *thrombophlebitis*, the intermittent application of moist hot packs is usually sufficient. In severe cases with fever, consultation with a physician should be sought, the arm kept in a sling and antibiotic and anticoagulant agents administered.

As mentioned, *allergic* reactions to local anesthetics may occur, although rarely. Whatever the offending drug may be the initial treatment for a fall in blood pressure is the administration of oxygen, followed, if necessary, by the intravenous administration of pressor drugs (see below under shock) and an adrenalcorticosteroid such as Decadron. Antihistamines such as diphenhydramine (Benadryl) are also to be administered parenterally (10 mg) followed by 50 mg given orally[13] three times a day. Subsequent analgesics should be of a different chemical structure.[1]

The prophylaxis[4] and treatment for *syncope, convulsions*, or *shock* consists in placing the patient in a horizontal position and administering oxygen, if necessary with intermittent positive pressure. If the convulsions do not cease when this method is employed, intravenous injection of a short-acting barbiturate such as pentobarbital or secobarbital sodium should be given, slowly, and in just barely enough quantity to stop the convulsion. Because barbiturates add to the depression which follows the convulsion, the administration of oxygen must be continued for some time. If the blood pressure has dropped and does not rise following this treatment, then a pressor drug such as mephentermine (Wyamine, 20 to 80 mg intramuscularly or 15 to 30 mg intravenously) or phenylephrine (Neo-Synephrine 2 to 5 mg intramuscularly or 0.2 to 0.5 mg intravenously)[13] should be administered. The rationale for the use of sympathomimetic drugs in the treatment of shock is questionable[7] (p. 515). Their use should be regarded as a temporary emergency measure. It has also been found that the intravenous administration of 100 mg of dexamethasone sodium phosphate U.S.P. (Decadron) is useful, and this treatment may be repeated if necessary.

Acute asthmatic attacks should be treated with epinephrine (0.25 to 1.0 mg given intramuscularly) or aminophylline given intravenously. When given intravenously to patients with severe obstructive dyspnea who are refractory to adrenergic compounds, Modell[13] suggests the intravenous injection of 250 mg of aminophylline in 10 ml of diluent. The drug should be injected slowly over a period of 10 minutes. Rapid injection may provoke a severe reaction or death. It may be that 150 mg will provide relief. If it is necessary to use the intramuscular route, then 500 mg is administered. To control the pain caused by this highly irritating drug, the injection of the aminophylline should be preceded by that of 2 per cent procaine solution without vasoconstrictor. The ampules of aminophylline are packaged for either intramuscular or intravenous injection, and care must be taken not to confuse them.

The prophylaxis for dental patients with *hypertension, cardiovascular*, or *cerebral disease* consists in control, by careful sedation, of the rise in blood pressure due to endogenous epinephrine.[5,11] Only light sedation is induced, but the elevated blood pressure reverts to the patient's usual level and does not subsequently rise after the use of local anesthetic solutions with vasoconstrictors and the surgical or restorative treatment. At Loma Linda University, dental patients with hypertensive, cardiovascular, or cerebral disease are always sedated because inadequate anesthesia resulting from a solution without epinephrine results in the pain-stimulated release of significant amounts of endogenous epinephrine, thus subjecting even the sedated patient to the risk of a hypertensive episode. It is recommended that great care be taken when administering local anesthetic solutions containing epinephrine to any patient who is taking a monoamine oxidase inhibitor. Our reading of the literature does not reveal a consensus as to the effect of the monoamine oxidase inhibitors.

Management of Toxic Reactions

Throughout this discussion it is stressed that we are dealing with potent drugs. Although there have been no serious side effects from these procedures in our experience since 1945, still one must always be prepared for a reaction. Fortunately, the depressive effects occur in the respiratory system before they become dangerous to the cardiovascular center. Thus there is a built-in safeguard. It would seem logical to use a pharmacological antagonist to a barbiturate-induced depression. However, at present no safe and efficient antagonist is available. For instance, pentylenetetrazol (Metrazol) in too large a dose will result in convulsions, and even a therapeutic dose which stimulates respiration will be followed by an equally deep depression. The consensus is that the remedy to use in case of respiratory depression is immediate ventilation with oxygen, using intermittent positive pressure if necessary.

If there is depression following the injection of meperidine, it can be counteracted by the use of oxygen followed by nalorphine given intravenously.

Toxic reactions to scopolamine and/or atropine are rare and do not involve anything more alarming than tachycardia and disorientation. They do not require treatment.

Serum hepatitis can be prevented by thoroughly cleansing and then sterilizing instruments which penetrate the soft tissues. Needles should be autoclaved at 121° C for 15 to 30 minutes, or by exposure to dry heat at 160° to 180° C for at least one hour. The sterilized article should not be stored in disinfecting solutions because such solutions may become contaminated with pathogenic microorganisms through careless handling. The Council on Dental Therapeutics of the American Dental Association further recommends the use of presterilized disposable hypodermic needles and syringes, as well as the employment of individual dose cartridges or ampules which, of course, should never be used for more than one patient.[1] The treatment of viral hepatitis rests with the physician, and fatalities following dental treatment are recorded.

SUMMARY AND CONCLUSIONS

Much patient distress during the administration of local anesthesia could be avoided by the use of 25-gauge, or heavier, short-bevel or Huber point needles (Fig. 4–2, page 38), aspirating syringes, or cartridges and the slow administration of minimum volumes of solution.

In the treatment of toxic or psychic reactions the administration of oxygen is usually the best method. No dental office is adequately equipped unless the dentist can immediately administer oxygen under pressure. If the patient does not recover rapidly, medical assistance should be summoned.

The spread of serum hepatitis can be prevented in the dental office by the use of sterilized needles and syringes and by never using a portion of any one anesthetic cartridge on more than one patient.

Finally, the best way to prevent local or systemic complications such as trismus, neuritis, cellulitis or phlebitis is to adhere strictly to the principles of asepsis and anatomy. An understanding of human physiology, coupled with a carefully taken history of the patient, can prevent complications ranging from mild allergy to total collapse.

BIBLIOGRAPHY

1. *Accepted Dental Therapeutics*, 33rd ed. Chicago, American Dental Association, 1969/70.
2. Adriani, John and Campbell, Donovan: Fatalities following topical application of local anesthetics to mucous membrane. Amer. Med. Assoc. J., *162*:1527, 1956.
3. Berlove, I. J.: *Dental-Medical Emergencies and Complications*. Chicago, Yearbook Medical Publishers, Inc., 1959, p. 128.
4. Bourne, J. G.: *Studies in Anesthetics: Including Intravenous Dental Anesthesia*. London, Lloyd-Luke Medical Books Ltd., 1967, Chap. 4.
5. Cheraskin, Emanuel and Prasertsuntarasai,

T.: Use of epinephrine with local anesthesia in hypertensive patients. IV. Effect of tooth extraction on blood pressure and pulse rate. J. Amer. Dent. Assoc. *58*:61, 1959.

6. Clutton-Brock, John: Two cases of poisoning by contamination of nitrous oxide with higher oxides of nitrogen during anesthesia. Brit. J. Anaesth. *39*:388, 1967. (See also Annotation in Lancet *2*, 930, 1967.)
7. Goodman, L. S. and Gilman, Alfred, eds.: *The Pharmacological Basis of Therapeutics*, 4th ed. New York, The Macmillan Co., 1970.
8. Harris, S. C.: Review of dental therapeutics, 1960. J. Amer. Dent. Assoc. *62*:502, 1961.
9. Jorgensen, N. B.: Measurements for intraoral block of the maxillary nerve. J. Oral Surg. *6*:1, 1948.
10. Jorgensen, N. B.: Accidental intravenous injection of procaine in dentistry. J. Southern Calif. Dent. Assoc. *20*:17, 1952.
11. McCarthy, F. M.: Clinical study of blood pressure responses to epinephrine-containing local anesthetic solutions. J. Dent. Res. *36*:132, 1957.
12. *Medical Letter on Drugs and Therapeutics. Interaction of Drugs.* New York, Drug and Therapeutic Information, Inc., *12*:93, 1970.
13. Modell, Walter, ed.: *Drugs of Choice, 1970/71.* St. Louis, C. V. Mosby Co., Chaps. 3, 14, 26 and 29.
14. *Physician's Desk Reference*, 24th ed. Oradell, N. J. Medical Economics, Inc., 1970.
15. Sicher, Harry and Dubrul, E. Lloyd.: *Oral Anatomy*, 5th ed. St. Louis. C. V. Mosby Co., 1970, p. 420.
16. Smith, A. E.: *Block Anesthesia and Allied Subjects.* St. Louis, C. V. Mosby Co., 1920, pp. 380–390.
17. SAAD: *Intravenous Anesthesia* (S. L. Drummond-Jackson, ed.), 4th ed. London, Society for the Advancement of Anesthesia in Dentistry, 1970.
18. Worth, H. M,; *Principles and Practice of Oral Radiologic Interpretation.* Chicago, Yearbook Medical Publishers, Inc., 1963, p. 212.

*Acknowledgment is made of the permission granted by W. B. Saunders Company to use a portion of this material which is adapted from The Dental Clinics of North America, November, 1965.

Chapter

6

A Method of Outpatient General Anesthesia for the Oral Surgical Patient

Adrian O. Hubbell, D.D.S., and R. Quentin Royer, D.D.S.

Over the last twenty-five years we have administered more than 10,000 general anesthetics a year by the methods next described and have noted a minimal number of complications.[1,2] This favorable experience is also reported by hundreds of dentists in the United States[3,4,5] and in other countries.[6,7] The administration of general anesthetics by dentists in their offices compares favorably for safety with the administration of general anesthetics in any hospital.[8,9,10]

EQUIPMENT AND PERSONNEL

In addition to the training and experience of the dentist, adequate equipment and able personnel are necessary. When these elements are all present and in readiness in a dental office, methods of general anesthesia will be utilized regularly and efficiently. Two or more dental chairs and one recovery room for each chair are desirable. Anesthesia equipment, surgical suction, oxygen, and nitrous oxide are required. The operator should have three assistants working with him as a team. A fourth assistant is most useful (Fig. 6–1). All ancillary personnel should be trained to assist with both the dental and anesthesia techniques. If necessary, dental procedures may be discontinued at any stage of the work and the complete team can devote their full attention to the anesthesia management. Greatly increased safety is assured the patient when four people, all trained in anesthesia techniques, work as a team. A recovery room nurse and receptionist are also needed. Thus, a minimum office staff of five assistants for one dentist is recommended. The experienced team will find great efficiency and ease in performing dental work by these methods.

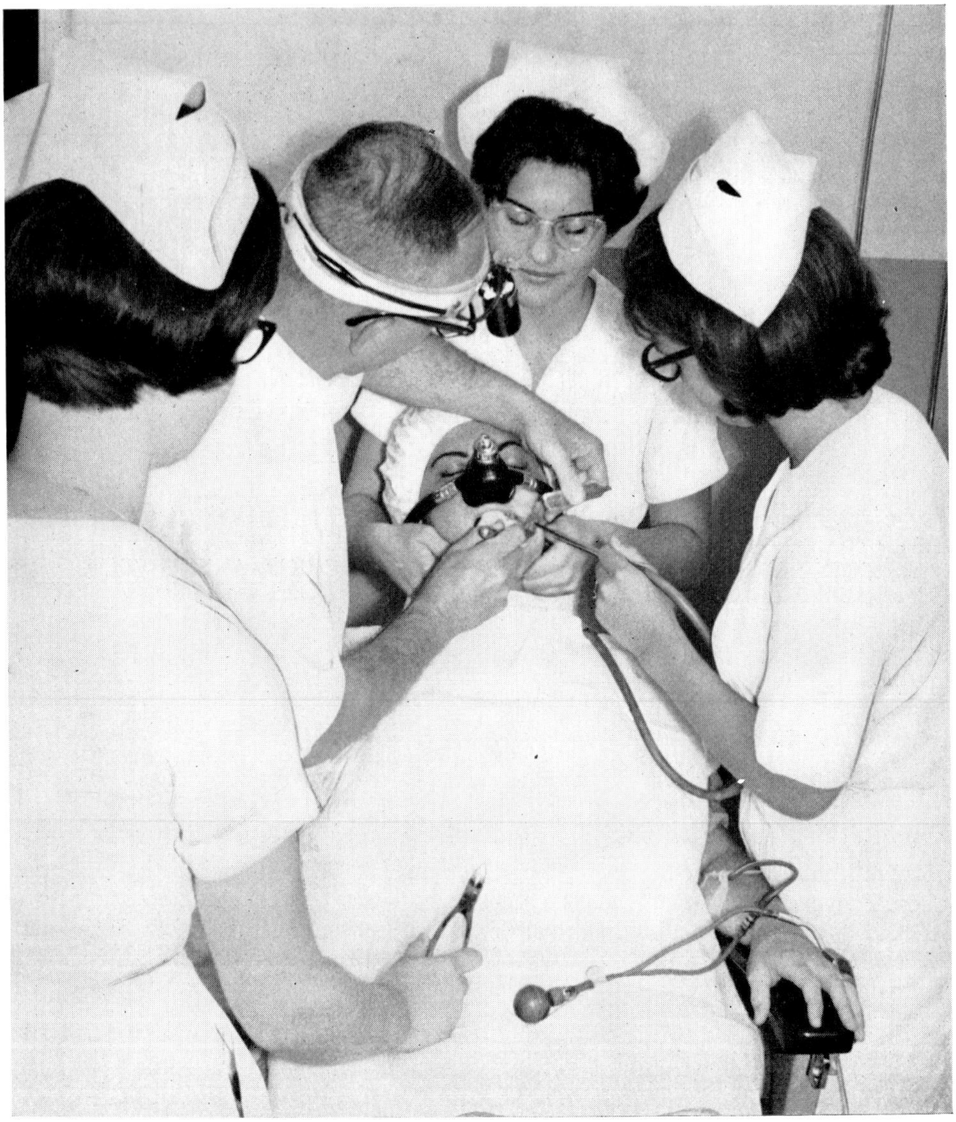

FIG. 6–1. Operative-anesthesia team. A minimal team of four expedites both anesthesia and dental techniques. Most dental procedures are managed best with the patient in the semireclining position.

TREATMENT PLANNING

The total dental treatment is planned as completely as possible before the appointment, and the amount of treatment to be done at any one appointment is left to the judgment of the dentist. Only the treatment which can be accomplished with complete safety and with reasonable effort on the part of the dentist and his team should be completed at one appointment. There is no contraindication to successive frequent appointments for the individual patient while utilizing this type of general anesthesia.

PATIENT SELECTION

The physical evaluation of the patient scheduled for general anesthesia is accomplished as outlined in Chapter 1.

There are increasing numbers of active people with heart disease. Most of these do well under general anesthesia. The patient who performs everyday physical activity without distress (dyspnea or chest pain) has a satisfactory functional reserve for general anesthesia. Edema of the ankles is frequently associated with impaired cardiac function and should be investigated; the ankle edema may be due to conditions which do not reflect an alteration in the cardiac reserve. The patient who is dyspneic at rest or orthopneic is not a suitable risk for general anesthesia. Any signs of cardiac decompensation should contraindicate general anesthesia for elective procedures. The patient in syncope or in shock from any cause should not be given a general anesthetic.

The doctor should observe the patient for age, weight, color, general vitality, and veins. Physical characteristics which affect the airway are important. Individuals with micrognathia frequently cannot breathe with the mouth open wide enough for dental treatment. This may be tested by having the patient bite on the child-size mouth prop. Ankylosis of the temporomandibular joint or inability to flex the cervical spine due to disease or injury should preclude office general anesthesia because these complications limit the access and control of the airway. The very obese frequently present airway problems.

PREOPERATIVE INSTRUCTIONS

The patient is instructed to avoid food or liquids for at least four hours before the dental appointment. A responsible adult must accompany the patient, who is instructed not to drive a car for four hours after the appointment. The nervous patient may be given pentobarbital sodium (50 to 100 mg) at bedtime the night before the appointment. For some apprehensive patients this medication may also be required one hour before the appointment time. Most patients, however, do not require it. Medications should be used only when a specific need is met by their use. When many different drugs or anesthetic agents are combined indiscriminately, it is difficult to determine the need for or the effect of the necessary drugs.

PREPARATION FOR ANESTHESIA

Everything necessary for the anesthetic and the operative procedures is ready at the appointed time. The patient is seated in the dental chair and draped. A deep reclining position is recommended. The blood pressure cuff and aspirator tubing are positioned. A sternal-notch stethoscope is helpful to monitor both the pulse and respiratory exchange simultaneously for most subjects. All drugs, equipment, materials, and instruments are at hand so that the procedures may be carried out without interruption. The patient's mouth is examined for prosthetic appliances, loose teeth, fragile crowns, or bridgework.

PRELIMINARY MEDICATION

The intravenous route of administration of premedicants is preferred. Premedication may be given five minutes before the anesthetic is started to allow full effect. It is not recommended for procedures requiring five minutes or less of anesthesia time. For longer procedures, atropine (0.4 mg) is recommended. Atropine is a depressor of the parasympathetic nervous system. Depression of the parasympathetic nervous system allows the sympathetic nervous system to dominate. This results in a higher metabolic rate, increased cardiac rate, and a decrease in oral and pharyngeal secretory gland activity. Diazepam (Valium) 2.5 mg to 10 mg given intravenously to effect a drowsy or heavy-eyelid level of sedation is most useful for some patients. Diazepam is a tranquilizing drug which depresses the central nervous system, reduces irritability, lowers the metabolic rate, lowers blood pressure and pulse, and facilitates the combined use of methohexital sodium and nitrous oxide and oxygen. Light levels of methohexital sodium cause an increase in blood pressure and pulse. The control of blood pressure during general anesthesia for the hypertensive patient is facilitated by diazepam. Diazepam is useful for patients who are resistive to light levels of methohexital sodium.

When the need for control of immediate postanesthesia pain is anticipated, fentanyl (Sublimaze) 0.5 mg, given intravenously at the start of anesthesia, is recommended. This potent narcotic gives effective postoperative pain control. Of all the available narcotics, this drug causes the least depression, hypotension and nausea. It may be used in combination with diazepam when indicated.

SELECTION OF ANESTHETIC AGENT

Methohexital sodium (Brevital) and thiopental sodium (Pentothal) are both excellent drugs and may be used alone or in combination with one of several of the inhalation anesthetic agents. Methohexital sodium is the agent of choice for the ambulatory patient. Its shorter action allows accurate control of depth of anesthesia by small intermittent doses. It eliminates prolonged recovery periods. Dental procedures of an hour or more are possible for the ambulatory patient when methohexital sodium is the principal anesthetic agent and no long-lasting premedication is used.

Both methohexital sodium and thiopental sodium provide a rapid, excitement-free induction and also have the advantage of an amnesic effect which permits many nonpainful procedures to be done when the patient is apparently awake. Therefore, no unpleasant postoperative memory ensues. The effect of any dose of methohexital sodium is brief so that the level of anesthesia may be adjusted as dictated by the stimuli to be covered. Painful procedures may be performed with light levels of anesthesia. Little respiratory depression is noted. The patient may be allowed to waken in a few minutes and the occlusion may be checked or nonpainful procedures performed. Methohexital sodium has little cumulative effect and recovery times for brief or long procedures are almost the same. The last patient of the day may be given an anesthetic for as long a time as necessary without keeping the office staff overtime. Diazepam premedication with methohexital sodium anesthesia does not prolong recovery time unduly.

INDUCTION

A vein of the forearm or antecubital fossa is selected and the venipuncture is made. The needle is attached to the arm with tape and the arm is restrained with a wrist strap (Fig. 6–2). As the induction dose of methohexital sodium is started, a mouth prop is inserted and oxygen is administered via nasal inhaler. Optimum results are obtained by the injection of 1 per cent methohexital sodium solution at the rate of 15 mg (1.5 ml) per second. The induction dose should provide a working level of anesthesia and the operation should be started as soon as the induction is complete. A mouth pack is placed to protect the pharynx from blood or foreign material.

The full effect of an induction dose of methohexital sodium is noted in twice the arm-to-brain circulation time, or about 30 seconds for the average adult.[11] When a

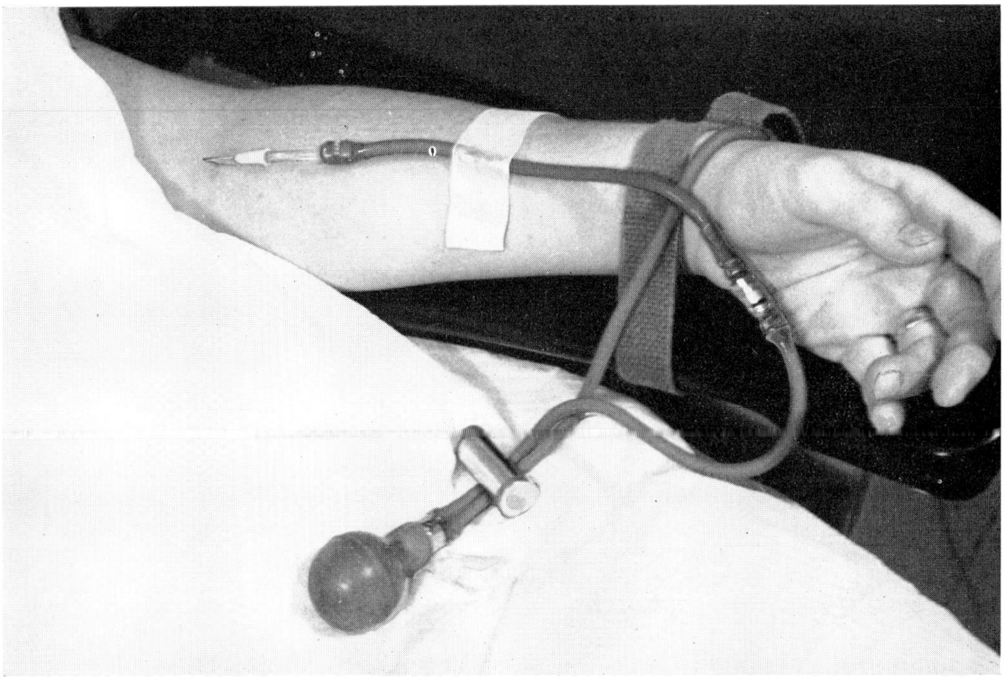

FIG. 6–2. Injection equipment. The needle is fixed to the arm with tape. The injector shown here eliminates the need for multiple syringes. Many excellent types of apparatus are available which allow successive injections and avoid the necessity of one of the team holding a syringe.

brief painful stimulus is to be covered (for example, a single extraction) and a minimum induction dose is desired, it is best to avoid stimulating the patient until the full effect of the induction dose is obtained.

DOSAGE

Dosage varies with age, vitality, and degree of apprehension of the patient. The debilitated and aged require less than do the younger or healthier subjects. The induction dose for a middle-aged adult in good health is about 80 mg (8 ml). The wild uncooperative 7-year-old child might require the same dose for complete induction. The frail 70-year-old patient might require no more than 20 mg (2 ml).

If the dosage is inadequate, jactitation will result, thus preventing a high-quality surgical result. Jactitation occurs because pain stimuli reach the brain, and can be prevented by the addition of N_2O or by the use of a local anesthetic.

MAINTENANCE

To maintain a working level of anesthesia it is necessary to make intermittent supplemental injections of one-third to one-half of the initial dose. The experienced dental anesthetist can anticipate the need for additional methohexital sodium; slightly increased muscle resistance to the mouth mirror or retractor and breathing changes are subtle indications. Swallowing is also a useful indicator to signal the need for additional methohexital sodium if painful procedures are to continue. A balance between anesthesia and the operative stimuli may be maintained as the procedure moves steadily

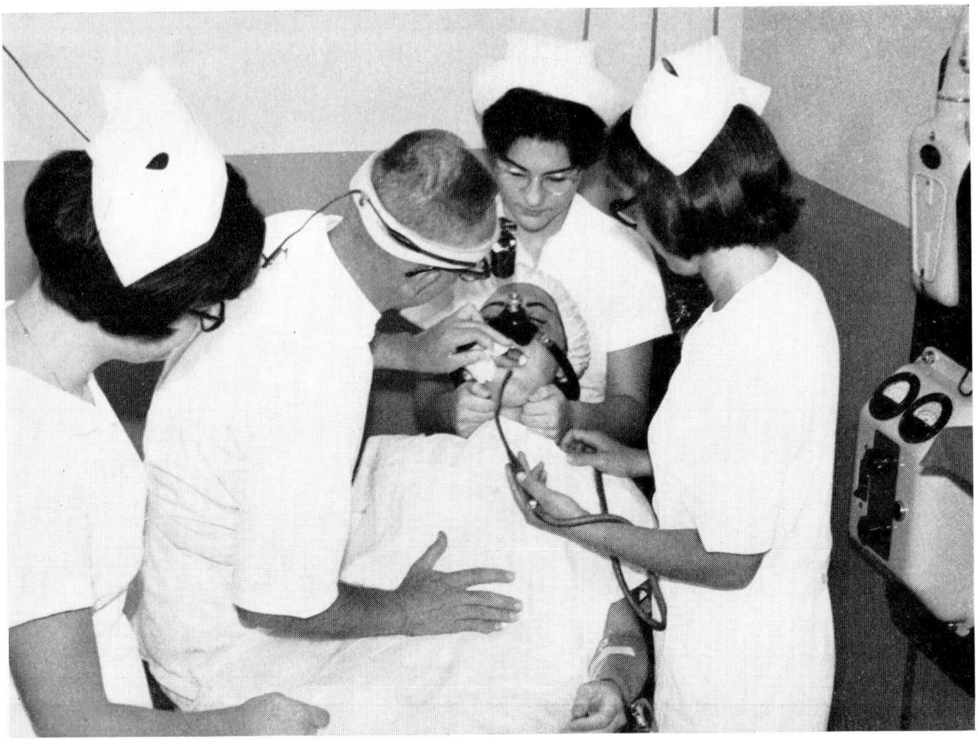

FIG. 6–3. A method of supporting the respiration manually with the patient's mouth open. Alternate compression of the lower rib cage provides adequate tidal volume.

ahead to completion. Maintenance of anesthesia by intermittent injections of methohexital sodium provides an up-and-down pattern of anesthesia depth. When these changes are extreme, the inhalation agents may be used to smooth out the pattern. Thus, the use of a supplemental inhalation agent such as nitrous oxide allows for greater time intervals between injections and decreased amounts of methohexital sodium.

This combination of methohexital sodium and nitrous oxide is not recommended for short procedures because several minutes are required for the patient to eliminate nitrogen from the lungs and anesthetic apparatus. Little benefit to the anesthetic procedure is gained until the greater percentage of nitrogen in the patient's system is replaced by nitrous oxide. Time as well as skill is required to pack the oropharynx to exclude all air from the system.

The oxygen supplied to the patient should never be less than 20 per cent. Some gas machines deliver less oxygen than the gauge registers, and it is common practice to compensate by maintaining at least 30 per cent oxygen on the anesthesia machine controls. This mixture of nitrous oxide and oxygen is not effective as a sole anesthetic agent for most patients. Used with methohexital sodium and given time for the nitrous oxide to replace the greater part of the nitrogen in the alveolar air and plasma, it is a valuable aid in maintaining a uniform level of anesthesia.

SUCCINYLCHOLINE CHLORIDE U.S.P.

Succinylcholine chloride is a most valuable agent for production of muscle relaxation. Light anesthesia, which is ideal for dental procedures, is sometimes complicated by partial or complete laryngeal spasm. Succinylcholine chloride in doses of 5 mg (for children) to 10 mg (for any adult) is specific for this complication.[12] It produces the desired effect in exactly the arm-to-brain circulation time (average 15 seconds).[14] After its administration, and prior to relaxation, the pharynx is examined for mucus, blood, or other irritants. These, if present, are removed.

Given in the doses recommended above, succinylcholine chloride rarely arrests the respiration. If respiratory arrest or depression occurs, the respiration may be manually supported by maintaining the patient's chin up, his tongue forward, and applying alternate pressure over his lower rib cage until adequate voluntary respiration is resumed (Fig. 6–3). This method is preferred to the use of an oral pharyngeal airway and the full face mask because access to the mouth and pharynx is possible while supporting the respiration.

RECOVERY

When the operative procedures are complete, the patient is observed in the dental operatory until all reflexes are active and he is responding to commands. Recovery time may be identified herein as that period between the completion of the dental procedure and the patient's intelligent response to commands. This is usually only *2 to 5 minutes*. Although patients who have been anesthetized are able to walk from the dental operatory in a few minutes, it is safer to transport them in a wheelchair to a recovery area where a nurse keeps them under observation. Weeping for a few minutes during the recovery room period is not uncommon following anesthesia produced by methohexital sodium. A stage of anxiety may occasionally follow methohexital sodium anesthesia; this should be differentiated from the crying jag which is usually terminated in 10 to 15 minutes and is not remembered by the patient. Anxiety, characterized by wringing of the hands, sleeplessness, and weeping, may last 24 hours or more. Compazine (10 mg) or pentobarbital sodium (50 mg) given intravenously provide effective treatment. Either drug may be taken orally every 6 hours after the patient has returned to his home if required to allay nervousness.

Patients should be dismissed only when they are completely steady on their feet. They should be accompanied to their homes by a responsible adult who has been informed that they will have impaired judgment and coordination for a period following the anesthesia.

The ability to drive a car safely after anesthesia has been studied by Wilkinson.[7] Following anesthesia produced by methohexital sodium, patients showed excellent performance after 10 minutes. There was no performance deterioration after 20 minutes. Factors which will alter the reaction time are: (1) the nature and dosage of drugs used for preliminary medication, (2) variable reaction of different patients to drugs, and (3) the length of anesthesia. These should be considered by the dentist when dismissing patients. A wide margin of time between anesthesia and driving a car should be prescribed.

ENDOTRACHEAL ANESTHESIA

The brief action of methohexital sodium and succinylcholine chloride makes the endotracheal method possible for the office patient. Although we prefer to hospitalize those patients for whom we believe endotracheal anesthesia is indicated, a number of dentists regularly use the endotracheal method of anesthetic administration in the dental office (Fig. 6–4).

The endotracheal method has several disadvantages. It requires a deeper level of anesthesia. Nasal or pharyngeal bleeding and laryngeal edema may result from the trauma inflicted by the endotracheal tube. Pain in regions of the skeletal musculature may result from succinylcholine when it is used in sufficient dosages to obtain the relaxation required for intubation. Longer

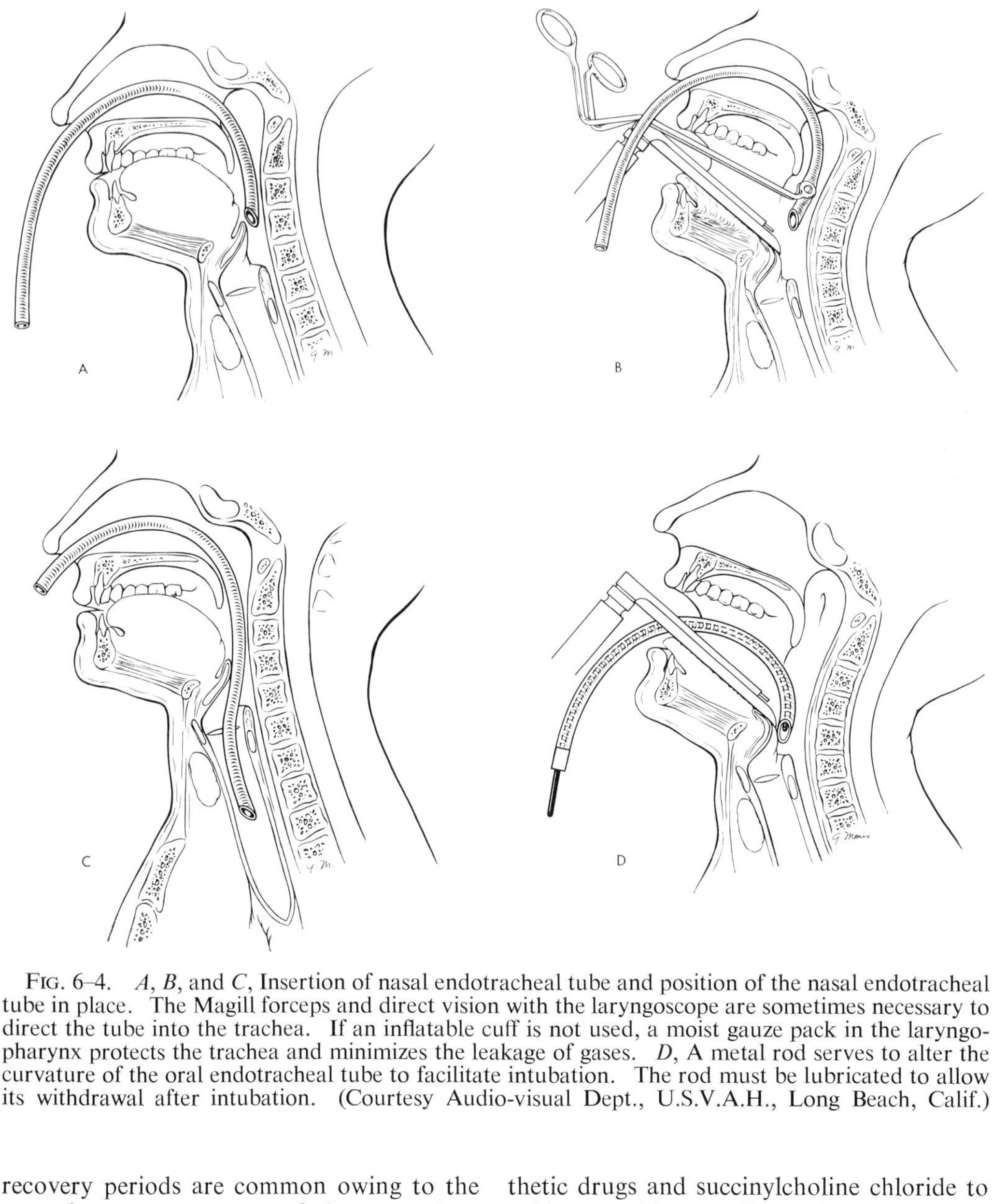

FIG. 6–4. *A*, *B*, and *C*, Insertion of nasal endotracheal tube and position of the nasal endotracheal tube in place. The Magill forceps and direct vision with the laryngoscope are sometimes necessary to direct the tube into the trachea. If an inflatable cuff is not used, a moist gauze pack in the laryngopharynx protects the trachea and minimizes the leakage of gases. *D*, A metal rod serves to alter the curvature of the oral endotracheal tube to facilitate intubation. The rod must be lubricated to allow its withdrawal after intubation. (Courtesy Audio-visual Dept., U.S.V.A.H., Long Beach, Calif.)

recovery periods are common owing to the use of greater amounts of drugs used to maintain the deeper levels of anesthesia. For some patients these disadvantages are minor when weighed against the advantages gained.

The advantages are: (1) more positive airway control, (2) controlled breathing, and (3) the ability to manage some resistant patients not manageable under light anesthesia. The occasional resistant individual who must be completely relaxed with anesthetic drugs and succinylcholine chloride to achieve working conditions for dental work will require intubation.

Nasal intubation is preferred to oral intubation because the presence of the tube in the oral cavity impedes the work of the dentist. The experienced anesthesiologist will rarely encounter greater difficulty inserting a nasal endotracheal tube than an oral one. When nasal intubation is difficult, the oral route can be used (Fig. 6–4*D*). Endotracheal anesthesia is conveniently done in the morning to allow for greater recovery time and longer postanesthetic surveillance.

After induction of anesthesia with methohexital sodium or thiopental sodium, relaxation is obtained with succinylcholine chloride given intravenously in doses of from 10 mg (for children) to 35 mg or more (for adults). The succinylcholine may be given by intravenous drip—0.2 per cent succinylcholine chloride solution in normal saline solution administered until relaxation is sufficient for intubation. The relaxation provided by succinylcholine chloride lasts a minute or more, giving time for insertion of the tube into the trachea and connection to the anesthesia machine. Manual control of respiration is started and succinylcholine chloride administration discontinued. A combination of nitrous oxide and oxygen (30 per cent) or oxygen and halothane (1 to 2 per cent on the Fluotec Vaporizer), as required to maintain anesthesia, is commonly used to supplement intermittent doses of methohexital sodium or thiopental sodium.

A one-way valve at the connection to the tube provides for a nonrebreathing technique which minimizes dead air space in the anesthetic apparatus (Figs. 6–5 and 6–6). Avoidance of dead air space is important in the anesthetic management of children in whom the respiratory tidal volume is small. Partial rebreathing is frequently used when nitrous oxide is employed as a supplement. Sufficient gases are allowed to escape to avoid excessive carbon dioxide in the system. Some anesthetists prefer a closed system in which no gases are allowed to escape and carbon dioxide is eliminated by absorption with soda lime.

An inflatable cuff near the tracheal end of the tube may be filled with a few cubic centimeters of air to make a positive seal. Some anesthesiologists prefer to pack the oral pharynx with a damp gauze pack, instead of

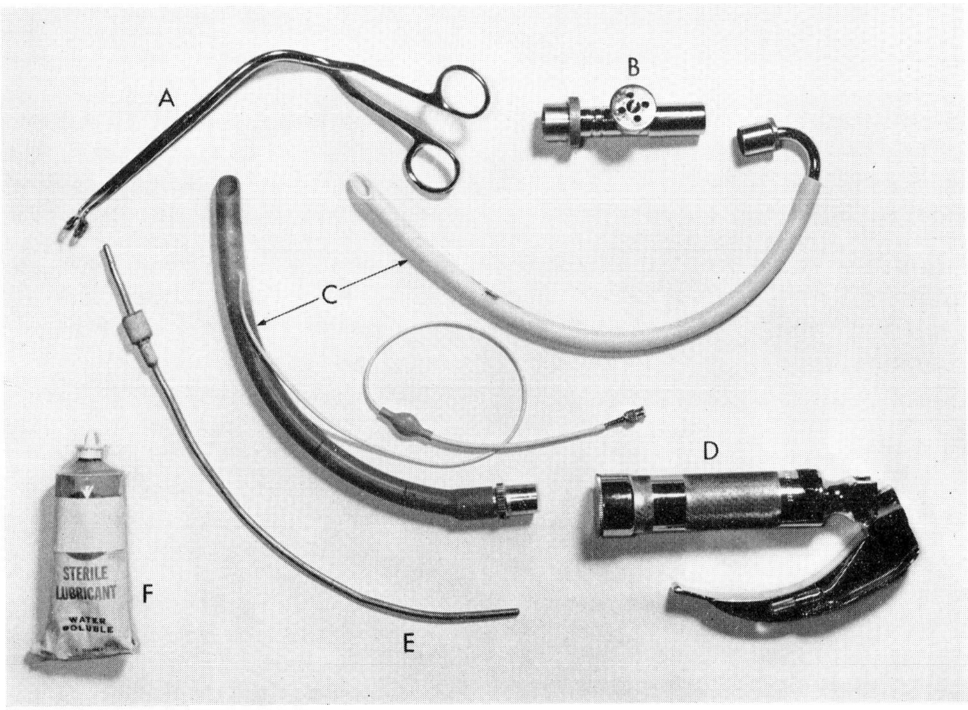

FIG. 6–5. Equipment for intubation. *A*, Magill forceps used to direct nasal endotracheal tube into trachea. *B*, One-way valve and connector from tube to gas machine tubing. *C*, Endotracheal tubes. *D*, Laryngoscope. *E*, Introducer to direct oral endotracheal tube into trachea. *F*, Lubricant for tubes and introducer.

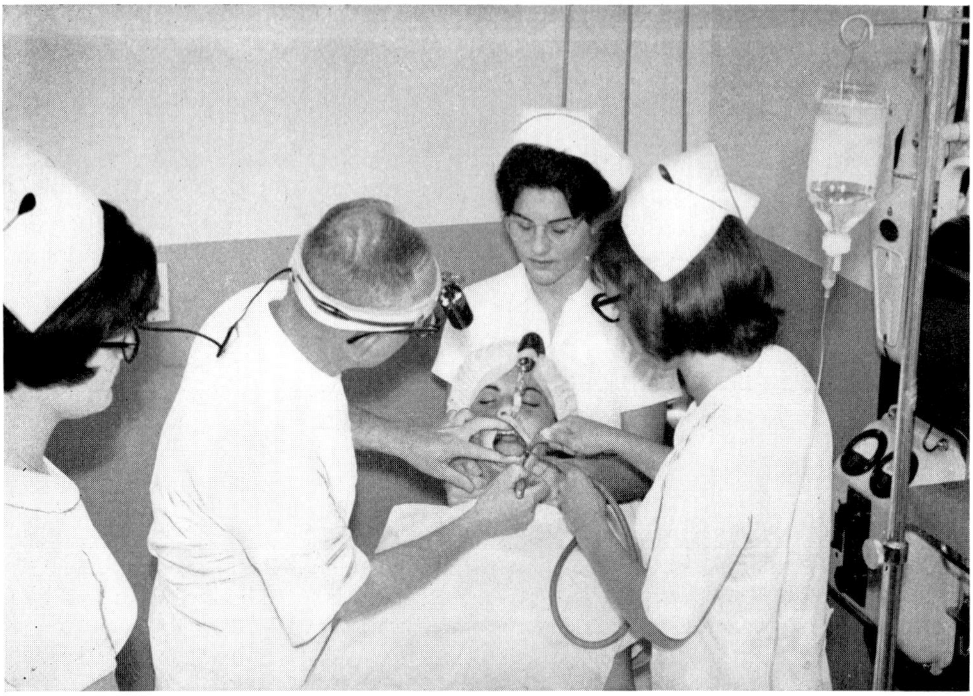

FIG. 6–6. Operative-anesthesia team with nasal endotracheal tube in place. A continuous drip of normal saline solution is used for longer procedures. It keeps the needle patent and serves as a vehicle for adding medications during anesthesia.

using the inflatable cuff. The gauze pack simplifies the removal of foreign material from the pharynx. At the end of the operation, administration of the anesthetic is discontinued and the endotracheal tube is left in place until the patient is sufficiently awake to cough. A suction catheter inserted into the endotracheal tube may be used to remove any excess secretions in or just beyond the tube. The pharynx is checked to make certain that it is free of foreign material or packs before the tube is removed.[13,14]

AGED AND DEBILITATED PATIENTS

The aged or debilitated patient has a much slower circulation time than does the younger or healthier subject. Smaller doses of the anesthetic given at longer intervals are indicated. The elderly or debilitated patient may be given oxygen for a few breaths, then 50 per cent nitrous oxide and oxygen for a preinduction period before the injection of a 20- to 30-mg (2 to 3 ml) dose of methohexital sodium. This combination, given in this order, allows procedures to be performed with the patient in a half-waking amnesic state with minimal changes in pulse, blood pressure, and respiration. The technique imposes less drug depression and, therefore, less physiological abuse for the debilitated than does anesthesia of greater depth. Slight occasional response to painful stimuli may be expected. Amnesia is complete and patients are uniformly pleased with the painless procedure. This technique is not satisfactory for the younger patient of greater general vitality.

Many monitoring devices are available which record the heart beat with a visual or an audible signal or both. None of these monitors relieves the dentist and his team of constant attention to good anesthesia management. General anesthesia requires an alert team, with continuous evaluation of the patient's status.

THE DENTAL ANESTHESIA TEAM

Why should a dentist devote much of his time and effort in order to master the science and art of general anesthesia as it pertains to dental treatment? The synchronization of general anesthesia and treatment, as has been described, necessitates implementation of each simultaneously with adjustments of each to accommodate the other. Thus, "the right hand must know what the left hand is doing." If the management of induction and maintenance of general anesthesia is delegated to someone other than the operating dentist, this may cease to be the case. For example, if anesthesia and treatment are not in harmony, the depth of anesthesia for the patient may be too great at certain stages of the procedure and too little at a critical stage of the operation. The cost would be prohibitive if, for every procedure, the patient would be asked to pay fees for the separate services of a dentist and an anesthesiologist. Too many patients need too many dental procedures to allow fees for both specialists to be economically realistic. By utilizing the methods described herein, the patient will benefit by having the best of both dentistry and anesthesia at reasonable cost.

BIBLIOGRAPHY

1. Hubbell, Adrian O.: Methohexital sodium anesthesia for oral surgery. J. Oral Surg. *18*:295, 1960.
2. Hubbell, Adrian O. and Royer, R. Quentin: Brevital sodium and pentothal sodium. Oral Surg., Oral Med., Oral Path. *16*:426, 1963.
3. Bullard, O. K. and Brockett, S. I.: Combined pentothal sodium-nitrous oxide-oxygen anesthesia in oral surgery. J. Oral Surg. *3*:138, 1945.
4. Krogh, Harold W.: Use of thiopental sodium in dental surgery. J. Oral Surg. *5*:337, 1947.
5. Millhon, J. A.: Pentothal sodium anesthesia for dental surgery in office practice. A review of 3,434 cases. Anesth. Analg. *29*:163, 1950.
6. Drummond-Jackson, S. L.: A milestone in intravenous anesthesia. Corresp. Brit. Dent. J. *113*:404, 1962.
7. Wilkinson, G. A.: Driving ability and reaction times following intravenous anesthesia. New Zeal. Dent. J. *61*:21, 1965.
8. Seldin, Harry M. and Recant, Benjamin S.: The safety of anesthesia in the dental office. J. Oral Surg. *13*:199, 1955.
9. Seldin, Harry M.: Survey of anesthetic fatalities in oral surgery and a review of the etiological factors in anesthetic deaths. J. Amer. Dent. Soc. Anesth. Feb., 1958.
10. McCarthy, Frank M.: Facts and fallacies regarding general anesthesia in dental offices. J. Oral Surg. *19*:492, 1961.
11. McCarthy, Frank M. and Hubbell, Adrian O.: Blood velocity in semirecumbent patients receiving ether, dehydrocholate sodium and thiopental sodium. J. Int. Anesth. Res. Soc. *36*:29, 1957.
12. McVeigh, John B. and Hubbell, Adrian O.: Succinylcholine chloride in oral surgery practice. J. Oral Surg. *17*:30, 1959.
13. Lundy, John S.: *Clinical Anesthesia.* Philadelphia, W. B. Saunders Co., 1942.
14. Cullen, Stuart C.: *Anesthesia in General Practice.* Chicago, Yearbook Medical Publishers, Inc., 1954.

Chapter 7

Educational, Economic and Social Aspects of Sedation and General Anesthesia

R. Quentin Royer, D.D.S., and Jess Hayden, Jr., D.M.D.

The purpose of this chapter is to consider in a general way the ways in which sedation or general anesthesia for the ambulatory dental patient can help to increase the delivery of dental health treatment. Mention will be made of certain educational philosophies and procedures which are believed to be important in the realization of this goal, and of the economic and social implications of the treatment.

THE PHILOSOPHY

General anesthesia for the ambulatory dental patient is a service for which there are particular indications, such as those for the unmanageable child,[5] the mentally and physically handicapped[9] and the candidate for oral surgery. If one considers the total population to receive general anesthesia, probably the largest numbers of patients requiring hospitalization will come from the first two categories. For those who can receive general anesthesia as outpatients, practical and safe methods in the office are used by many oral surgeons and increasing numbers of general practitioners. Surveys of record have shown that the administration of general anesthetics by dentists in their offices compares favorably for safety with the administration of general anesthetics in any hospital.[7,8] McCarthy reports dental office general anesthesia to be safer than hospital general anesthesia for minor surgery: "I should like to stress the fact that a comparison of death rates after general anesthesia administered in oral surgery offices with general anesthesia death rates in hospitals is not done with the intention of placing medical anesthesiology in a poor light. It is unfair to compare such statistics without stressing the basic differences between the two. These differences acount for the great variation between office general anesthesia mortality and hospital general anesthesia mortality, a ratio which I place conservatively at 1:20. For example, office oral surgery procedures requiring anesthetics are purely elective and are performed on favorable risk patients, anesthetic duration is comparatively short, the surgery is relatively minor for the most part and rarely can become a threat to life, the surgery can be terminated rapidly if necessary, and operative delays are rare. All of these points of difference add greater hazards that are unavoidable to operations performed under general anesthesia in hospitals."[3]

Ambulatory anesthesia means that the patient comes to the dental operating suite, undergoes a state of general anesthesia during which time a surgical procedure is accomplished, and afterward regains consciousness and returns home to rest. This procedure differs from hospital anesthesia in that no long-lasting preoperative medications are given. The lightest plane of anesthesia consistent with pain control is recommended because, if anesthesia is maintained with the gag and cough reflexes present, there is greater protection against the inspiration of foreign material such as mucus, blood, or debris than is the case when these reflexes are absent. Ambulatory anesthesia allows for a more rapid return to consciousness and relatively normal postoperative activity for the patient.

The dental general anesthesia-surgical team is the key to this accomplishment.[1] The team should consist of the surgeon, a nurse to support the chin, a nurse to retract tissue and aspirate, and a nurse to pass instruments to the surgeon (Fig. 6–1). Each must be well trained and capable to understand both the general anesthesia and the surgical procedure. Each must be able to recognize emergency problems as well as to prevent them. In emergency situations the entire team must exhibit ability to function simultaneously for resuscitation of the patient. Utilization of intravenous barbiturates such as methohexital in conjunction with inhalation agents such as nitrous oxide is common practice. Atropine should be given as preliminary medication in longer cases except when contraindicated (glaucoma may be such a contraindication). The intravenous agent should then be administered in order to produce a relatively light state of surgical anesthesia. It will be noted that when this intravenous agent, methohexital, is given a very slight degree of apnea is noted. The pulse rate will be increased slightly or markedly with an increase in blood pressure. There are many patients, particularly the apprehensive ones in the teen-age range, who will require the addition of an analgesic agent. Nitrous oxide 50 per cent and oxygen 50 per cent adequately serve this purpose for some patients; in others, premedicating agents may be required. Intermittent doses of methohexital as described by Hubbell and Royer[2] should be administered until the surgical procedure is completed.

Usually the ambulatory anesthesia patient is not premedicated prior to coming to the office nor is he intubated during anesthesia. Obviously of great economic benefit is the fact that general anesthesia for the ambulatory patient does not require beds for preoperative sedation, and the post-anesthesia recovery time in the office is short.

There are physiological and pharmacological reasons why general anesthesia for the dental patient has enjoyed greater success in the office of the oral surgeon than in that of the general practitioner. The non-intubated patient, carried in a light stage of anesthesia, is not completely quiet and tends to move slightly during the procedure. Surgery can be accomplished well even if the patient has a tendency to move. Restorative procedures upon teeth, on the other hand, need to be so accurate that they are difficult to perform under the same conditions of patient movement; therefore, the patient must be brought to a deeper plane of general anesthesia. The bevelling of a cavosurface angle or the placing of a point angle in a gold-foil preparation are examples of the need for extreme accuracy in restorative instrumentation. For such work local anesthesia (Chap. 4) supplemented by inhalation or intravenous sedation (Chap. 3) is the method of choice. Local anesthesia with sedation provides an additional benefit, the patient's ability to cooperate with the dentist during treatment.

EDUCATIONAL REQUIREMENTS

Progress in control of anxiety, fear and pain will be directly proportional to its inclusion in the dental curriculum. The basic health sciences must be taught not only in the classroom and laboratory but also in the dental clinic, by dental faculty. Such exposure must be greatly expanded. Classic textbook exercises will be of no avail if the sciences are not applied to the patient. It is obvious that control of pain, with its base in anatomy, biochemistry, microbiology, pathology, pharmacology and physiology, is a subject which can meaningfully and effectively integrate these preclinical health sciences with clinical experiences. For example, within the field of physiology, the cardiovascular and respiratory components are of great importance not only during normal function but in the ever-increasing numbers of the ambulatory medical risk patient. Patients suffering cardiovascular disease must be appropriately managed. The risk patient can be monitored continuously by oscilloscope, but such mechanical monitoring means little unless the dentist has the knowledge of basic body function to couple with the monitor's output.

Gaseous interchange, vital to life and essential for inhalation anesthesia, must be understood. Mechanical obstruction to such interchange necessitates an understanding of anatomy. Both the chemistry and physics of such interchange belong in the curriculum.

Information relative to pharmacodynamics should be patient-oriented and related to drugs used to control anxiety and pain or to produce general anesthesia. The dentist must be able to apply this information both to normal healthy patients to prevent morbidity and to the already morbid. Both groups are increasing in number. The percentages of our population aged under 25 and over 65 attest to this.

Action of various drugs on heart rate and stroke volume are examples of the knowledge necessary for the dentist responsible for administration of sedation or general anesthesia. The level (depth) of sedation or anesthesia must be maintained so as not to depress the patient who is hypertensive and concomitantly taking antihypertensive medication. Depression is accompanied by hypotension, which must be avoided.

One concept of the core curriculum now under discussion in educational circles is that students in the health professions (dentistry, medicine, nursing, pharmacy, and graduate) be given an integrated core curriculum in preclinical health science. That is, during the first year they will take identical courses, and only after that move into their respective disciplines. For dental students, in-depth studies will occur during the clinical period of dental education. They first will be given the opportunity to observe faculty members who have demonstrated proficiency in the art and science of control of anxiety, fear and pain; they will be required to understand that physical diagnosis and the evaluation of the patient are built on the academic background of the sciences mentioned above: physiology, pharmacology, anatomy, biochemistry, physics, and microbiology. This period will also provide the beginnings of clinical practice under strict faculty supervision and will enable the student to acquire skill in establishing rapport, administering local anesthetics, and giving inhalation and intravenous sedation. It will provide a good foundation for later acquiring skills in general anesthesia, but will not provide adequate experience for administering general anesthesia. Those who need to acquire such expertise (for example, most oral surgeons) will need greater exposure to both clinical and academic experiences during a later period of residency. For the postgraduate interested in general anesthesia, Royer and Lundy[6] recommend as a beginning approximately six months spent in the operating room providing general anesthesia for all types of surgical cases, this to be followed by six months of training in ambulatory general anesthesia and surgery under the guidance of a dentist expert in both.

Educational experience in the accomplishment of ambulatory anesthesia can provide the skills associated with instantaneous decision-making, as illustrated by the need for the almost reflex judgments required to institute resuscitation procedures. Our dental schools need to move these principles into clinical practice, in order that the dental graduate will have had first-hand experience and participation in managing any ambulatory patient in case of emergency. Training beyond the professional degree must utilize and broaden experience with these methods. Nearly every hospital center should have a facility for providing outpatient ambulatory general anesthesia and inhalation or intravenous sedation.

Dental educators and organized dentistry must devote concerted effort to bring an understanding of these problems to the allied health professions, mainly medicine. Our allied health professions must assist in this important project of providing pain-free dentistry, because the multidisciplinary educational approach to health care is extremely important to the patient. The disciplines—all phases of medicine, dentistry, nursing, and pharmacy—*need to work together* within hospitals. Office facilities should be available where oral health care, both preventive and therapeutic, is available with all other facets of health care.[4] The patient should be able to travel to a "one-stop" ambulatory treatment, diagnostic, and preventive health center—a hospital, if you will—where he can reach the several disciplines of health care without traveling many blocks or miles to each. Obviously, this statement applies to all areas of health care, and is not limited to dental care.

ECONOMIC AND SOCIAL ASPECTS

The delivery of dental health care at a moderate cost to as many people as possible is the responsibility of our profession. A primary reason that dental treatment is not as universal as it should be is the attitude of the patient's family, friends, neighbors and the news media (particularly publications), all of which may frequently and adversely affect—that is, tend to frighten—the individual who needs treatment. Harrison Evans (Chap. 2) deals with certain common anxieties of the patient. The dentist in practice would more likely enumerate the factors affecting both the patient and the nonpatient as social, educational, and economic. There is much interplay between these factors and anxiety. Social, educational and economic factors require interdisciplinary approaches to solutions, and cannot always be resolved by the dentist and his staff. On the other hand, control of pain is one of the most important factors to be considered, and the dentist in his own office certainly can positively and with assurance control pain.

The control of anxiety, as Harrison Evans points out, begins with obtaining the patient's confidence through an attitude of "consideration, deliberation and deft assurance" on the part of the dentist (page 18). "Words are, of course, the most powerful drugs used by mankind," Kipling is reported to have said. Relatively simple psychotherapeutic techniques accompanied by local anesthetics (Chap. 4) supported when necessary by inhalation or intravenous sedation (Chap. 3) will undoubtedly control most of the imagined and real pain associated with dental practice, usually at a cost much less than that incurred with general anesthesia.

When general anesthesia is indicated, the favorable economics of outpatient general anesthesia should be given careful review. Physicians or other health-care personnel frequently recommend hospital general anesthesia on an inpatient basis for dental treatment. Often these well-meaning health professionals, and their patients, are unaware that the expense of such treatment may not be covered by third-party insurance. For example, the hospitalization charges for oral surgery or restorative dentistry, including the prolonged treatment period under general anesthesia, usually will not, at this writing, be paid for under third-party health insurance programs. Conversely, a relatively short and simple procedure such as myringotomy, and, of course, all longer general surgical operations under general anesthesia, usually will be paid for in part or in whole by third-party insurance. In certain geographical areas the routine cost of preoperative and postoperative bed care (24 to 36 hours total) and operating room and anesthesia charges will amount to several hundred dollars, to which must be added the dentist's fee. The major portion of the total cost is, therefore, related to the cost of hospitalization, and in many cases the patient would be better served on an ambulatory basis with a saving of time and dollars for all involved.

An understandable, but nonetheless real, problem is the matter of scheduling time for the use of the hospital surgical operating room. Dental treatment, except in hospitals with sufficient operatories and a good orientation to dental health needs, is often lowest on the priority scale of the day's operating-room schedule. That means that a session scheduled at 1:00 p.m. may not be started until 3:30 p.m. or later, and can involve a real waste of the dentist's time. The pressing need for the delivery of dental health care requires us to broaden our use of reasonable and safe alternatives to general anesthesia in the hospital operating-room suite. These alternatives have been discussed, particularly in Chapters 3, 4 and 6.

SUMMARY

Reduction of emotional stress upon patients will lead to more widespread health care. The undergraduate education of dentists must include the theoretical and practical experience that prepares a dentist to control pain in the dental office. All disciplines concerned with the delivery of health care must work together to impress upon the public that dental care can be accomplished without great emotional or financial stress. The development of dental offices within health-care centers will initially serve as a proving ground in accomplishing this goal, and can also provide a more realistic educational background for dentists and auxiliaries.

Anesthesia or inhalation and intravenous sedation combined with local anesthesia for surgical or restorative procedures are perfected to the point that every American could benefit from them *if the dental profession could be persuaded in adequate numbers to master the skill and knowledge to provide this care.* Professional education and a practice proving ground will be the approach to these endeavors and have been discussed under appropriate headings. Although research will provide yet unknown methods to lessen patient stress, adequate methods are now at hand and ready to be utilized on a broader base. Dental schools, hospitals and other health centers should avail themselves of them.

BIBLIOGRAPHY

1. Hagen, J. O. and McCarthy, F. M.: General anesthesia for the ambulatory patient; the anesthetic team. J. Southern Calif. Dent. Assoc. *37*:244, 1969.
2. Hubbell, Adrian O. and Royer, R. Quentin: Brevital sodium and pentothal sodium. Oral Surg., Oral Med., Oral Path. *16*:426, 1963.
3. McCarthy, Frank M.: Facts and fallacies regarding general anesthesia in dental offices. J. Oral Surg. *19*:492, 1961.
4. Royer, R. Q.: Hospital dentistry. In *Current Therapy in Dentistry*, Vol. 4. St. Louis, C. V. Mosby Co., 1970, pp. 455–457.
5. Royer, R. Quentin, and Hubbell, Adrian O.: *Current Therapy in Dentistry*: Oral Surgical Procedures for Children. St. Louis, C. V. Mosby Co., 1964, p. 577.
6. Royer, R. Quentin, and Lundy, John S.: The training of dentists in the field of general anesthesia. Amer. Dent. Soc. Anesth. Apr. 1957.
7. Seldin, Harry M.: Survey of anesthetic fatalities in oral surgery and a review of the etiological factors in anesthetic deaths. J. Amer. Dent. Soc. Anesth. Feb., 1958.
8. Seldin, Harry M. and Recant, Benjamin S.: The safety of anesthesia in the dental office. J. Oral Surg. *13*:199, 1955.
9. Sprague, Boyd: Controlled rectal anesthesia for the fearful or handicapped patient. J. Oral Surg. *16*:201, 1958.

Section III

Anatomy, Neurophysiology and Pharmacology

Chapter 8

Anatomy

The dentist or physician is particularly concerned with the facial anatomy when a patient experiences or anticipates unpleasant or painful sensation in the mouth or face. Then the cause of, or the route of transmission of, or the proper means of interruption of, unpleasant stimuli becomes a matter of immediate importance. Dentists routinely administer local anesthetics to interrupt unpleasant stimuli from the teeth, gingiva or soft tissues during restorative or surgical procedures and, perhaps less frequently, to encourage hemostasis, inhibit gagging, aid in differential diagnosis, or palliate facial pain. Certainly anatomy plays a large role in many dental treatments, although it is easy to lose sight of the three-dimensional relationships of the concerned connective tissue, vascular and nervous structures. Demonstrably, it is possible to operate with fair success within anatomical boundaries which the dentist does not recognize, but which are not to be transgressed without unpleasant after-effects. The purpose of this short review is to consider some anatomical structures related to the nervous elements important to local anesthesia in dental practice.

SUPERFICIAL MUSCLES, NERVES AND VESSELS

The more superficial structures to be considered in approaching the face from the oral vestibule are the mucosa; the muscles of facial expression with their fascial covering, particularly the levator anguli oris and levator labii superioris muscle; the facial artery and vein and the infraorbital nerve terminal branches (Fig. 8–2).

The levator anguli oris muscle arises immediately beneath the margin of the infraorbital canal, in the canine fossa, and inserts into the angle of the lip; overlying it is the levator labii superioris muscle arising from the maxilla and zygomatic bone and inserting into the upper lip (Fig. 4–17). Between the two muscles is a potential space filled with areolar connective tissue in which are found terminal fibers of the infraorbital nerve, facial

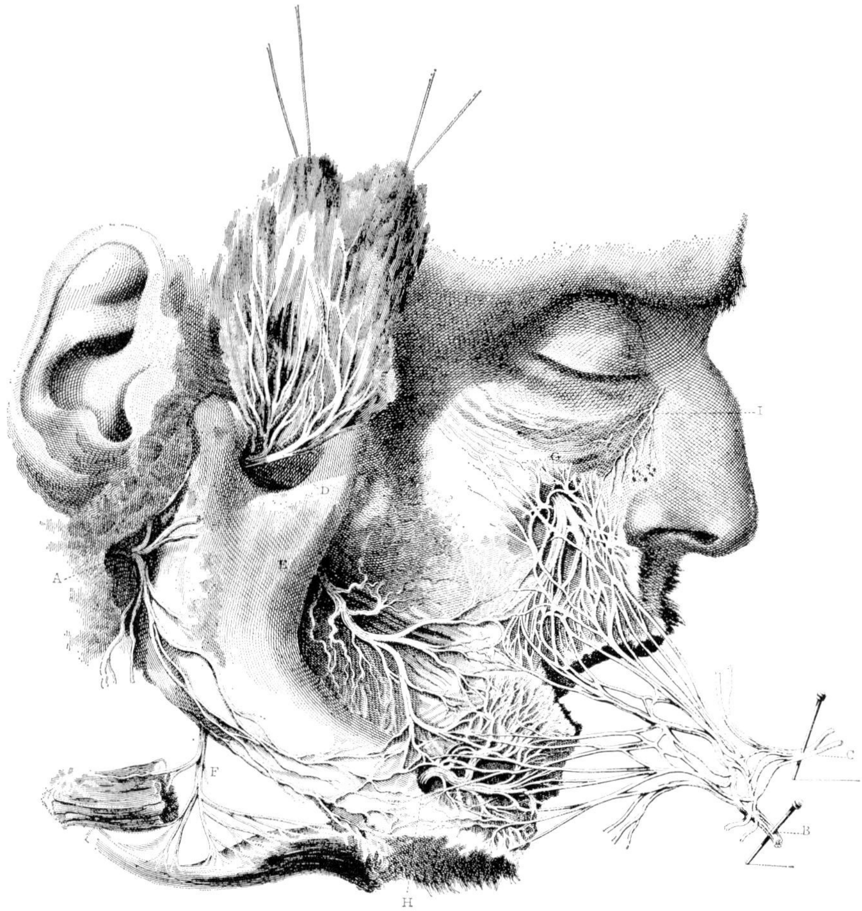

FIG. 8–1. Sir Charles Bell, in his 1829 paper on the nerves of the face, provided this representative drawing of certain sensory and motor fibers of the trigeminal nerve, fibers of the facial nerve, and a joining of some of the fibers of both nerves. (From Charles Bell: On the nerves of the face; being a second paper on that subject. Philos. Trans. Roy. Soc. London, p. 328, 1829.)

vein and sometimes the facial artery just before it enters the substance of the levator labii superioris alaeque nasi at the wing of the nose (at other times the facial artery lies on the levator labii superioris). The facial vein originates as the angular vein at the medial margin of the eye and relative to the artery follows a straighter course across the face, receiving numerous tributary veins. Its termination is in the common facial vein, which drains to the internal jugular vein (Fig. 8–2). The facial vein has no valves. Through the superior ophthalmic vein it communicates with the cavernous sinus, and by way of the deep facial vein with the pterygoid plexus. The anatomical course of the facial vein has direct relevance to clinical practice: an intravascular injection may easily occur where the facial vein lies behind the facial artery, and the area of the facial vein around the nose and upper lip is frequently called the "danger area" of the upper face. Infections in this area, although usually localized, may spread into adjacent vessels with the potential risk of thrombosis of the facial vein or even the cavernous sinus.

The pulse of the facial artery in the face is first detected on the base of the mandible, or a little above it, and anterior to the masseter muscle (Fig. 8–2). Here the artery is covered

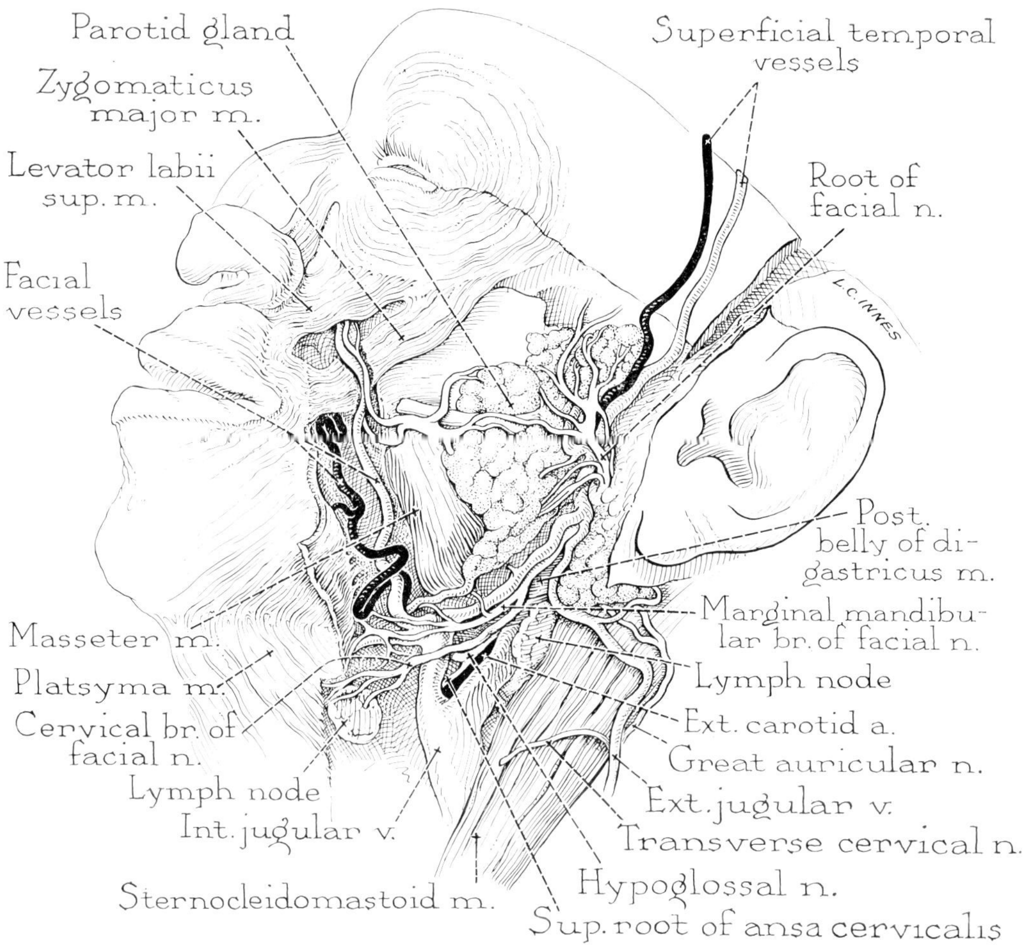

FIG. 8–2. Superficial dissection of face and neck structures. A window has been made in the zygomaticus major to show the course of the facial vein and one of the branches of the facial nerve. The parotid duct has been cut. (Courtesy W. H. Roberts, M.D. Reprinted from first edition.)

only by the platysma muscle, superficial fascia and skin. If there is a pronounced swelling in the area, the artery may be elevated into the buccal vestibule. As it nears the same horizontal plane as the commissure of the lips, the facial artery lies in the muscular mass contributing to the modiolus (Fig. 8–2) close to the mucous membrane of the lip; its pulsing may be felt from the oral cavity, permitting the dentist to monitor the pulse without removing his hand from the mouth. The inferior and superior labial arteries are its two branches on the face and it terminates as the angular artery. The facial portion of the artery has many convolutions.

Superficial nerves of the face involved in administration of local anesthetics include branches of the infraorbital, mental and facial nerve. The first two usually intentionally are anesthetized at their respective foramen. The latter is sometimes inadvertently anesthetized by a misplaced inferior alveolar injection after the nerve emerges from the stylomastoid foramen and approaches the posteromedial surface of the parotid gland.

The fascia covering the muscles of facial

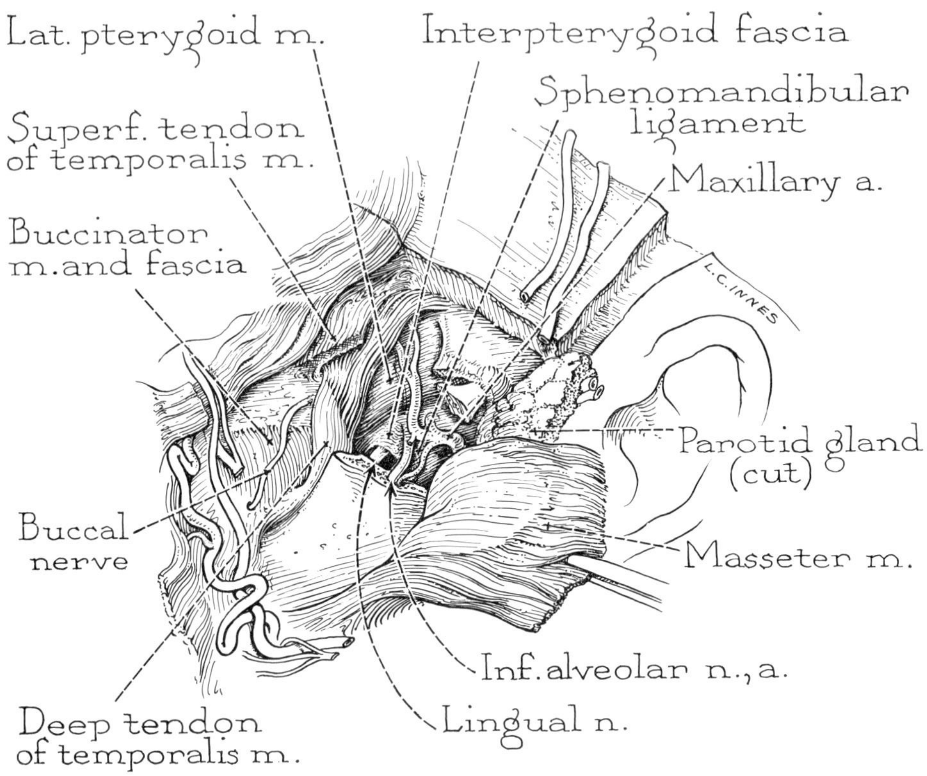

FIG. 8–3. Same specimen as drawn in Figure 8–2. Deep dissection shows relationship of inferior alveolar and lingual nerves to the interpterygoid fascia (the sphenomandibular ligament is the thickened posterior part of this fascia); the inferior alveolar nerve is lateral, the lingual nerve medial (a window has been made in the interpterygoid fascia to show the latter). (Courtesy W. H. Roberts, M.D. Reprinted from first edition.)

expression is not continuous, as it is in the neck, on the parotid gland, or covering the temporal and masseter muscles. For this reason, and because of the different levels of attachment of the various facial muscles, air or infection introduced by or following injections or other dental procedures may follow several routes. Worth[15] mentions air in the cheek following the hypodermic injection of a local anesthetic and documents six cases of surgical emphysema of the face due to various causes. Sicher's and Dubrul's[12] discussion of "The Propagation of Dental Infections" provides the dentist with an understanding of the process.

In summary, the hypodermic administration of a local anesthetic in the anterior region of the face should call to memory not only the bony skeleton but the relation of the facial artery and vein, terminal branches of the infraorbital and mental nerves, and the muscles of facial expression. Posteriorly, the masseter muscle and parotid gland and their fascia must be considered.

INFRATEMPORAL FOSSA

The region of the infratemporal and pterygopalatine fossae is important in regard to dental block anesthesia. The reward of an understanding of the spatial relationship and contents of these fossae is an enhanced ability to produce immediate and profound anesthesia and to reduce significantly the possibility of inadvertent injury caused by the improper positioning of a needle within the spaces.

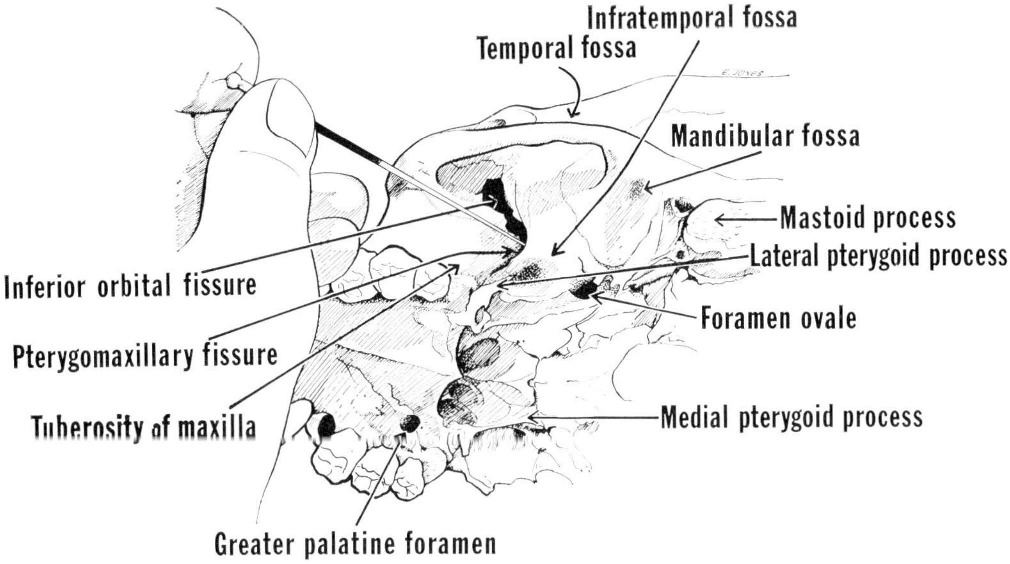

FIG. 8–4. The temporal and infratemporal fossa from an inferior and lateral view.

The irregular space of the infratemporal fossa (Fig. 8–4), as approached during a block injection from the buccal vestibule, may be described as extending upward to the infratemporal crest of the sphenoid bone, posteriorly from the tuberosity of the maxilla to the mastoid and styloid processes, and inward from the ramus of the mandible to the lateral pterygoid plate. The fossa has no anatomical floor and is variously described as having its inferior border at the alveolar margin of the maxilla,[14] or as continuing downward into the neck.[10] The importance of the fossa can be judged by its major contents, which are: the medial and lateral pterygoid muscles between which pass a portion of the maxillary artery and the pterygoid venous plexus as well as mandibular, inferior alveolar, lingual and chorda tympani nerves; the sphenomandibular ligament and communication with the inferior orbital fissure; the pterygomaxillary fissure, and the temporal fossa (Fig. 4–20).

MUSCLES OF MASTICATION; MASTICATOR SPACE (Fig. 8-5 A-C)

The four muscles of mastication and their associated vessels and nerves lie in the masticator space. The masticator space is enveloped by the upward extension of the cervical fascia, which passes between and over the surfaces of the temporal, masseter and pterygoid muscles to form an enclosed space.[14] The enveloping effect of the fascia is seen in Figure 8–5*c*.

The three muscles of mastication most likely to be pierced by a needle during deep injections in this area are the lateral and medial pterygoid muscles and the temporalis muscle at its tendon of insertion (Fig. 4–36). The insertion is mainly on the anterior portion of the inner plate of the ramus (Fig. 8–5*c*) and extends down to the area of the mandibular third molar as seen in Figures 4–36 and 4–39. In the latter figure the tendon lies just posterior to the needle tip. The superficial tendon can be palpated as it lies along the ramus, and particularly in the area of the coronoid notch (Figs. 4–30 and 4–31). It, therefore, is a reliable and helpful landmark in determining the plane of insertion of the needle (see The Injection, page 71). The tendinous lower portion of the muscle is forced against the maxillary

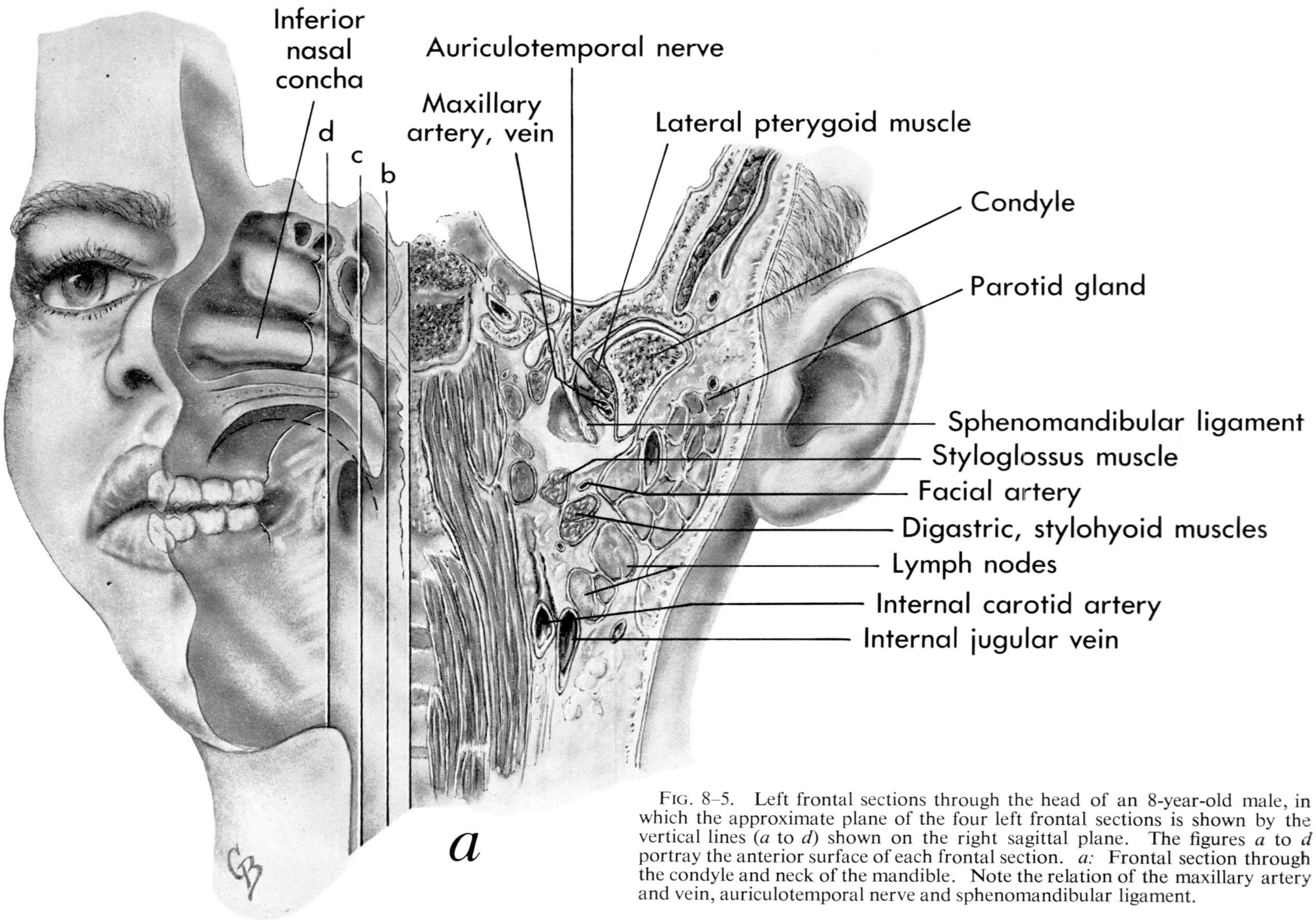

FIG. 8–5. Left frontal sections through the head of an 8-year-old male, in which the approximate plane of the four left frontal sections is shown by the vertical lines (*a* to *d*) shown on the right sagittal plane. The figures *a* to *d* portray the anterior surface of each frontal section. *a:* Frontal section through the condyle and neck of the mandible. Note the relation of the maxillary artery and vein, auriculotemporal nerve and sphenomandibular ligament.

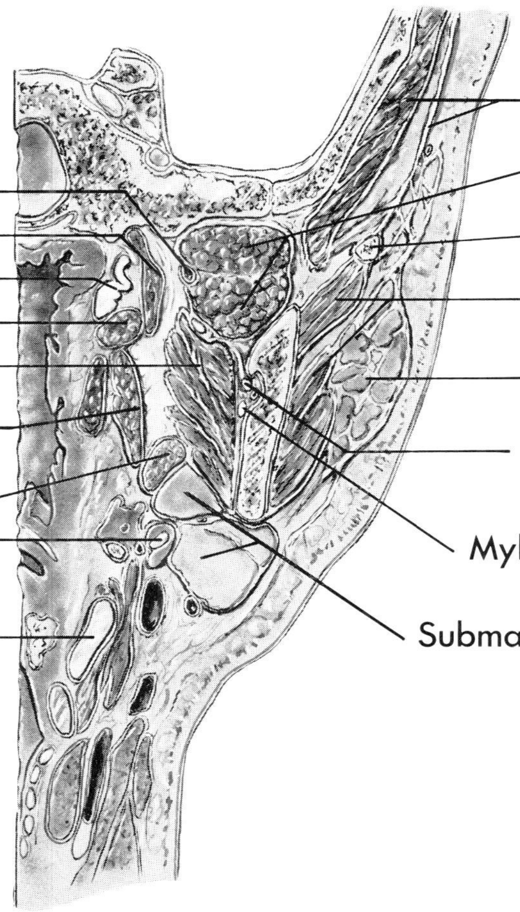

FIG. 8–5. *b:* Frontal section through the mandibular ramus at the mandibular foramen.

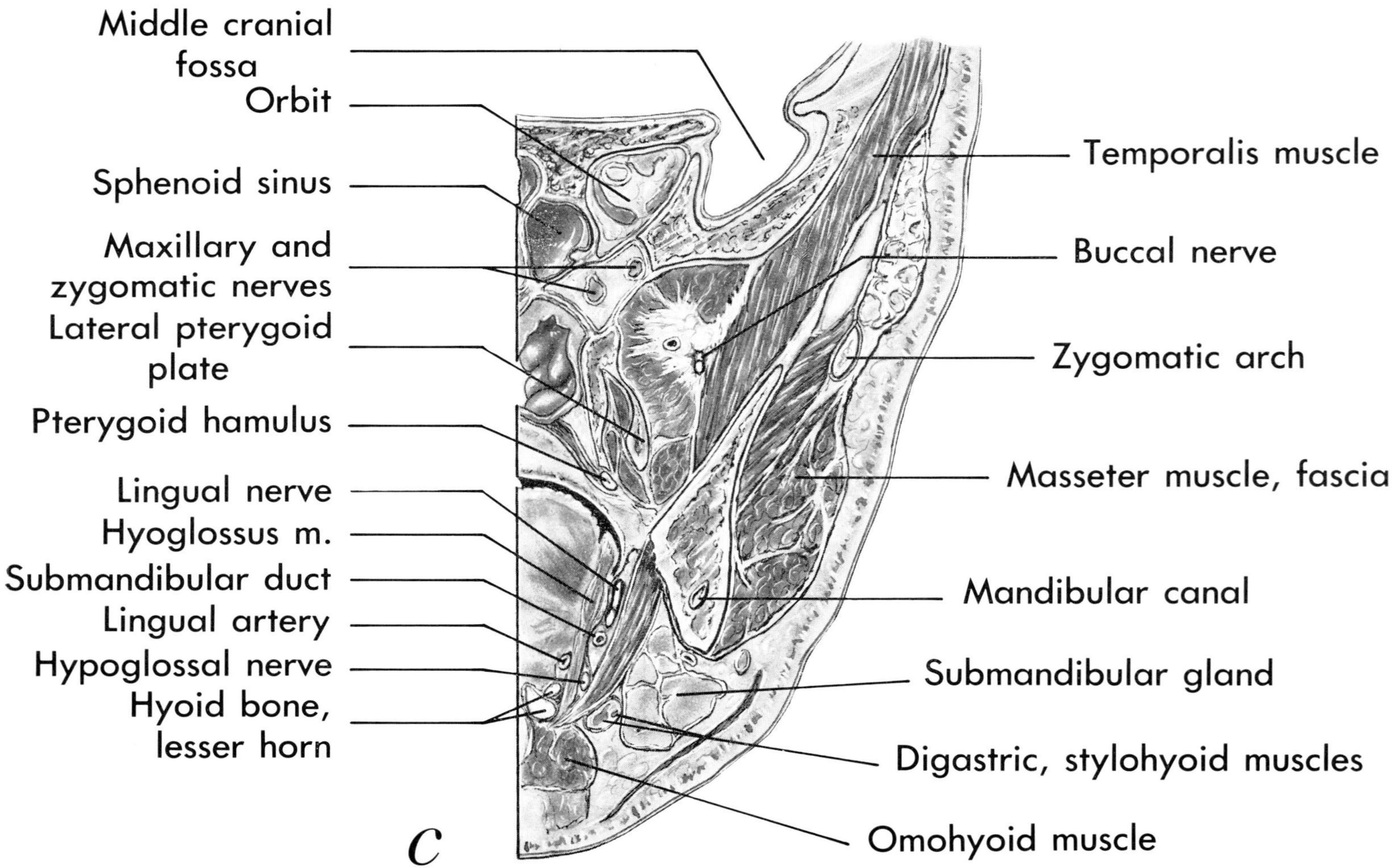

FIG. 8–5. *c:* Frontal section through the plane of the lesser horn of the hyoid bone and the pterygoid hamulus.

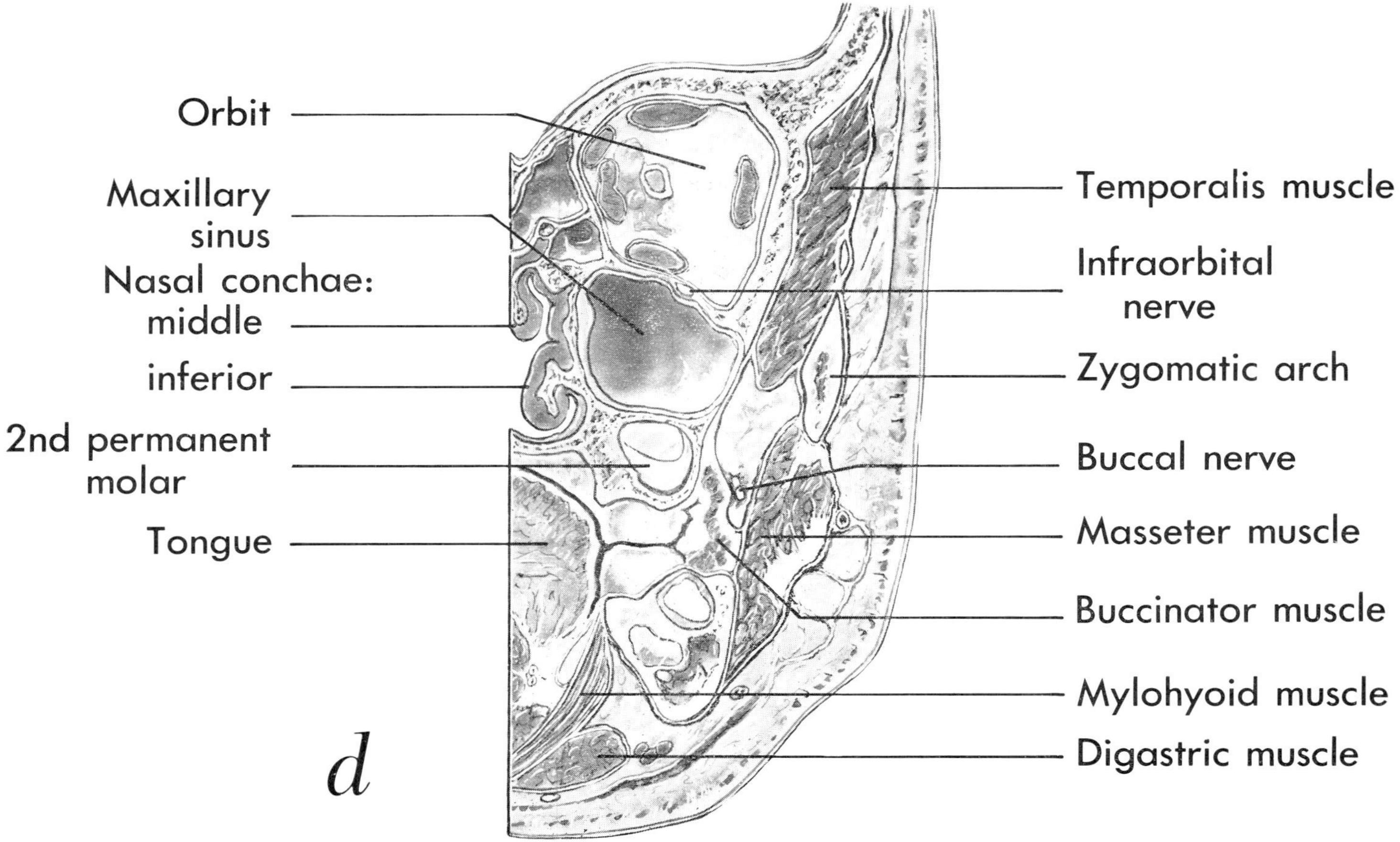

FIG. 8–5. *d:* Frontal section through the mesial surface of the unerupted 2nd permanent maxillary molar.

tuberosity when the mouth is wide open, making it difficult to perform a posterior superior alveolar block.

The lateral pterygoid muscle is often considered to lie too superiorly to be traumatized during injections. Actually, its position within the masticator space places it within easy striking distance of needle tips during posterior superior alveolar or inferior alveolar injections (Fig. 8–5*b*). The two heads of the muscle arise from the infratemporal surface (upper head) and lateral pterygoid plate (lower head) and insert by a common, short, thick tendon into the condyle, disc and capsule of the temporomandibular articulation.

The medial pterygoid muscle also arises by two heads. The smaller inferior head springs from the tuberosity of the maxilla and pyramidal process of the palatine bone, while the larger mass originates from the medial side of the lateral pterygoid plate and the depth of the fossa between the two plates. As seen in frontal section (Fig. 8–5*b*) fibers of the medial pterygoid muscle approximate the lower border of the lateral pterygoid muscle. From these origins the medial pterygoid muscle obliquely passes posteriorly, inferiorly (45°) and laterally to attach to the angle of the mandible. On the mandible the oblique groove for the mylohyoid artery and nerve lies just anterior to the muscle attachment, and so the vessel and nerve pass between the muscle and the mandible (Fig. 8–5*b*). The groove and roughened area of muscle insertion are visible in Figure 4–30.

The masseter muscle is situated on the lateral extremity of the masticator space (Fig. 8–5*b–d*). It arises from the zygomatic arch and its fibers pass down and backward to insert in a wide area in the region of the angle of the mandible and forward. The muscle is not directly involved in the usual approaches for dental local anesthesia, but in case of trismus its action in closing the jaws makes intraoral injections much more difficult.

The muscles of mastication are innervated by branches from the mandibular nerve trunk or its anterior division. Thus, if it is necessary to relieve trismus, these motor nerve fibers as well as the sensory components can be blocked by an extraoral approach to the foramen ovale (Mandibular Nerve Block, page 77).

PTERYGOPALATINE FOSSA

The pterygomaxillary (pterygopalatine) fissure (Figs. 4–20 and 8–4), a landmark well known to dentists through the study of cephalometric radiographs, marks the lateral entrance to the pterygopalatine fossae. The outline of the small fossa may be compared to an inverted trangle, with the skull for its base (Fig. 4–27*C*). It lies anterior-posteriorly between the posterior surface of the maxilla and pterygoid process of the sphenoid and laterally-to-medial between the pterygomaxillary fissure and the vertical plate of the palatine bone.

The fossa is the key to important and interesting anatomical relations. For instance, on the skull a probe can be passed successively through the infratemporal fossa, pterygomaxillary fissure, pterygopalatine foramen, sphenopalatine foramen and into the nasal cavity. Foramina on the posterior wall of the fossa include the pharyngeal, pterygoid canal, and rotundum which transmits the maxillary nerve. On the medial wall the sphenopalatine foramen transmits the sphenopalatine artery and the nasopalatine nerve, as well as other branches from the pterygopalatine ganglion and maxillary nerve. Below, the greater (major) palatine canal transmits descending palatine vessels and the palatine nerves (Figs. 4–27 and 8–6). The canal ends at the greater palatine foramen (Figs. 4–12 and 4–13) which the dentist familiarly approaches from the palate a little anterior to the pterygoid hamulus, and always in the same sagittal plane (Fig. 8–6).

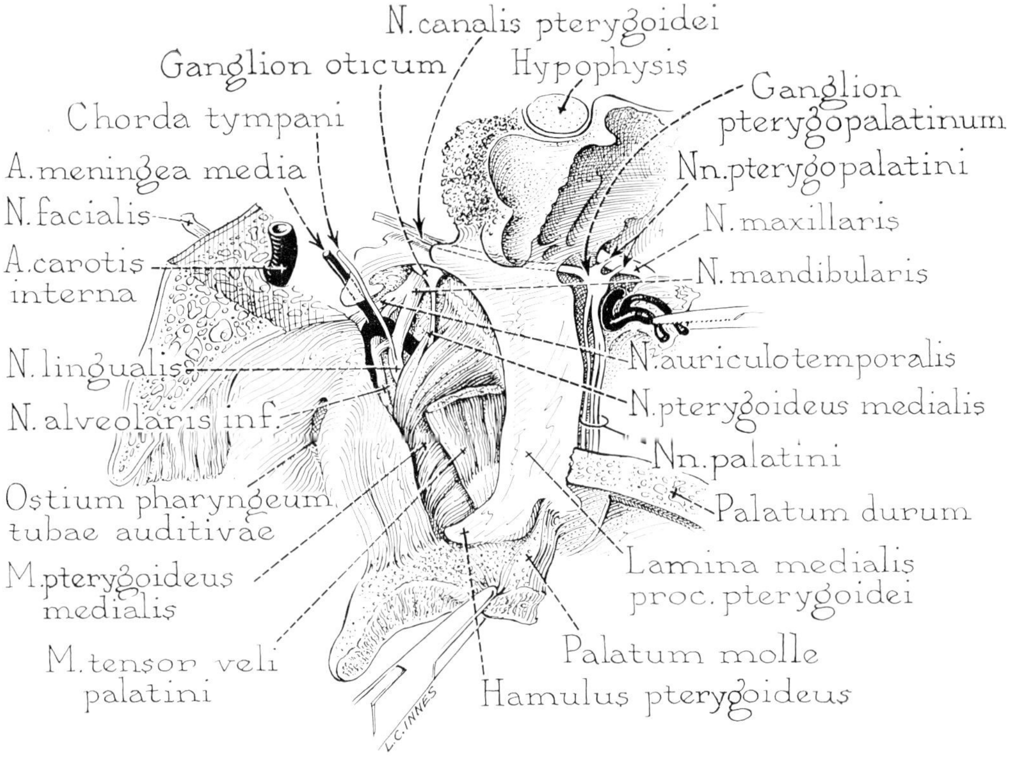

FIG. 8–6. Medial view of a dissected specimen sectioned in the midsagittal plane. It shows the mandibular nerve, its branches and the otic ganglion in the infratemporal region, and the maxillary erve, its branches and the pterygopalatine ganglion in the pterygopalatine fossa. (Courtesy W. H. Roberts, M.D. Reprinted from first edition.)

NERVES, ARTERIES, VEINS AND THEIR BRANCHES AND TRIBUTARIES

A description of the nervous and vascular system is classically designed to simplify for the sake of memory and clinical application the profuse network of nerves and vessels existing in the facial region. The facial nervous network was long ago examined by dissection and graphically or verbally described in the literature (Fig. 8–1). More recently, Bassett[2] published a monumental *Stereoscopic Atlas of Human Anatomy.* One section of the *Atlas* not only discloses the nerves but also provides some idea of the very generous blood supply of the head and neck.

The facial region is reflexogenous by about 8½ weeks of fetal life,[8] and the peripheral nervous system at the third month of fetal life exhibits the main branching found in the adult. Thus during fetal life the trigeminal nerve, for the most part, has developed the relationships which are characteristic of its course in infant, child and adult life, a point which should be remembered when administering local anesthetics to a child (Fig. 8–7). Surprisingly, innervation of the pulps of teeth, according to experimental evidence, may not occur until about the time of their eruption. The fifth nerve is the largest and one of the most complicated of the cranial nerves. It is the main sensory nerve for the skin of the face and anterior scalp, teeth, mouth and nasal cavity (general somatic afferent, exteroceptive and also proprioceptive from muscles) and the motor nerve to several muscles including the muscles of mastication (special visceral efferent). Of particular clinical interest is the fact that the trigeminal nerve is known for its examples of referred pain from other body areas or nerves; for exam-

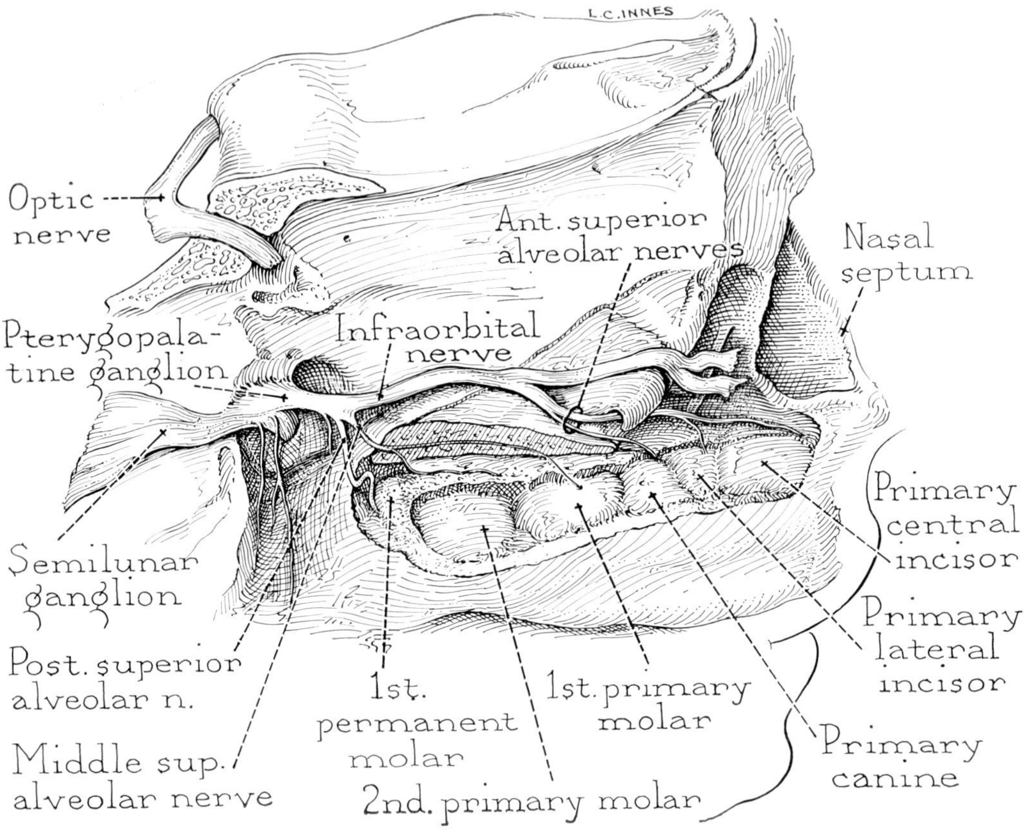

FIG. 8–7. Dissection showing the innervation of the maxillary teeth in an 8-month human fetus.

ple, irritation in one division of the trigeminal may be experienced as pain in another, or in the upper cervical, glossopharyngeal and vagus nerves.

Arising from the lateral side of the pons, the roots of the trigeminal nerve pass forward into the middle cranial fossa and form the trigeminal ganglion. The ganglion has three divisions: the ophthalmic, the maxillary and the mandibular. The first two divisions are entirely sensory, the third has sensory and motor components. The ophthalmic nerve will not be discussed in this text.

The direct sensory maxillary nerve leaves the skull through the foramen rotundum and enters the pterygopalatine fossa. There it breaks into three major branches: the internal represented by the pterygopalatine nerve, the intermediate by the infraorbital nerve, and the smallest and most external branch by the zygomatic nerve.[12] A number of its branches will be described in connection with the pterygopalatine ganglion (page 124).

The mixed sensory and motor mandibular nerve is the largest nerve of the infratemporal region. It enters the infratemporal fossa through the foramen ovale immediately posterior to the upper part of the lateral pterygoid plate (Figs. 8–4 and 8–6). Here the tensor veli palatini muscle separates the trunk from the auditory tube, while the lateral pterygoid muscle is on the lateral or superficial side. These muscular relations can be seen in Figure 8–5*b* in which the nerve trunk lies just behind the frontal plane of the section. The mandibular nerve trunk is only 2 to 3 mm in length. The trunk divides into an anterior division which is largely motor to the muscles of mastication, and a posterior division which is largely sensory through its auriculotemporal, inferior alveolar and lingual branches. The mandibular nerve, and thus its motor and sensory components, can be blocked at the foramen ovale (Fig. 4–44).

Facial and Maxillary Veins; Pterygoid Venous Plexus

The main arteries of the face are the facial and the two terminal branches of the external carotid artery, the temporal and the larger maxillary artery. The photographs of corrosion casts provide some idea of the extent of the facial vascular supply (Fig. 8–8). The superficial course and relations of the facial artery and vein previously were discussed (page 112). The venous return from the face is usually superficial with the *facial vein* as the chief vein receiving tributaries corresponding in general with all branches of the facial artery. The facial vein communicates with the cavernous sinus through the superior ophthalmic vein and with the pterygoid plexus through the deep facial vein. The *maxillary vein* corresponds to the first part of the maxillary artery, described below. The maxillary vein receives blood from the pterygoid plexus and joins the superficial temporal vein to form the retromandibular vein. The *pterygoid venous plexus* lies between the temporalis and the lateral pterygoid muscles, or the lateral and medial pterygoid muscles, according to the path of the maxillary artery. The tributaries of the plexus correspond with and accompany the branches of the maxillary artery; among them are the nasopalatine, pharyngeal, infraorbital, posterior superior alveolar, descending palatine, inferior alveolar, and buccal branches, and veins from the muscles of mastication, meninges and pterygoid canal. The venous drainage of the teeth arises from a rich plexus under the odontoblastic layer and passes to the named regional veins. The pterygoid plexus has both deep and superficial communications. For example, the plexus communicates with the cavernous sinus and the facial vein. The venous drainage of this area is tremendously complex; for details and further references, the interested reader should consult one or more of the regional or systematic anatomy texts listed in the Bibliography.

Maxillary Artery

Both the temporal and maxillary arteries are first deep to or embedded in the parotid gland. Immediately below the level of the neck of the mandible the maxillary artery arises and in its anterior course immediately enters the infratemporal fossa. For purposes of description its course has been divided into three parts: before, on, and beyond the pterygoid muscles or, respectively, mandibular (1st), pterygoid (2nd) and pterygopalatine (3rd) portions. As can be seen from the cross sections (Fig. 8–5) the artery is vulnerable to damage from needles at certain points in its path through the fossa. In its mandibular portion it lies between the neck of the mandible and the sphenomandibular ligament (Fig. 4–36). The auriculotemporal nerve lies above and the maxillary veins beneath (Fig. 8–5*a*). The artery, in this (1st) portion, between sections shown in Figure 8–5*a* and *b*, lies on the medial pterygoid muscle and the inferior alveolar nerve. The relation of the artery to the lateral pterygoid muscle is seen in Figure 8–5*b*, but the inferior alveolar nerve is obscured. In the pterygoid (2nd) portion it passes forward on the medial (usually lateral) surface of the lower head of the lateral pterygoid (Fig. 8–5*b*) and finally in the third or pterygopalatine portion enters the pterygopalatine fossa between the two heads of origin of the lateral pterygoid muscle (Fig. 4–23).

Inferior Alveolar Artery

The maxillary artery in the mandibular (1st) portion has five branches, two to the meninges, two to the ear, and one, the inferior alveolar artery, which runs downward to the mandibular foramen between the vein (behind) and inferior alveolar nerve (anterior) (Figs. 4–34 and 8–3). The artery runs forward in the mandible supplying the pulps of the teeth, the bone of the mandible and its periosteum and gingiva. The mental artery arises at the mental foramen to supply

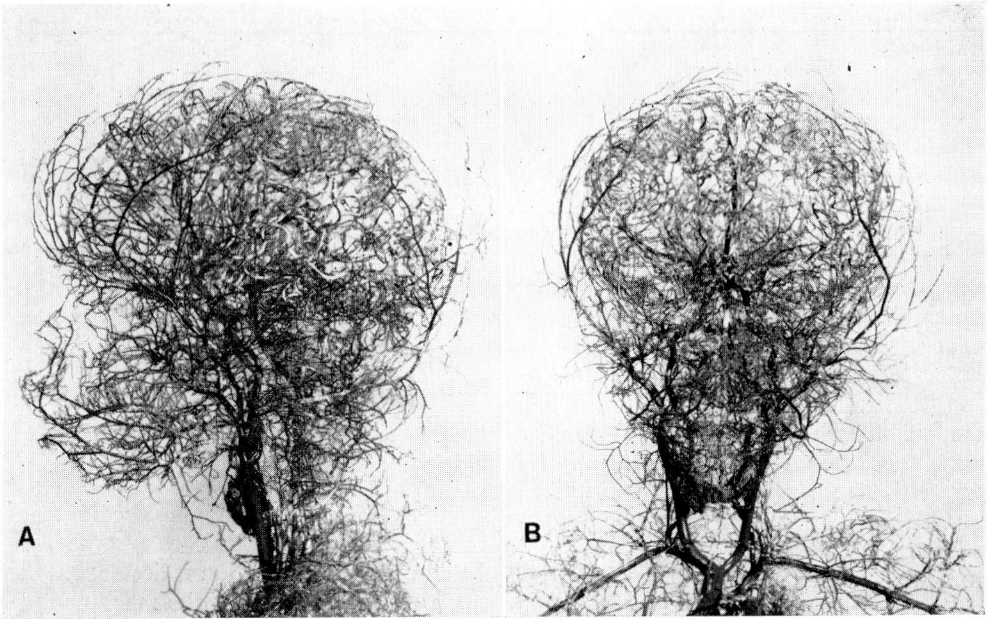

FIG. 8–8. Photographs of part of a corrosion cast of the arteries of the head and neck of a stillborn baby. *A*. Left lateral view. *B*. Anterior view. (Courtesy of the Wellcome Museum of Anatomy and Physiology of the Royal College of Surgeons of England, × 1/2.)

the nearby skin and muscles while fibers from the parent trunk continue anteriorly to supply the incisor teeth.

The five arterial branches of the pterygoid (2nd) portion, with their accompanying veins, are the buccal and those to the four muscles of mastication.

The branches of the pterygopalatine (3rd) portion are the posterior superior alveolar artery, infraorbital artery, artery of the pterygoid canal, descending palatine artery, sphenopalatine artery and pharyngeal artery. The first two of these arise before the maxillary artery passes through the pterygomaxillary fissure to the pterygopalatine fossa and divides into terminal branches. The size of the posterior superior alveolar artery is such that it easily may be damaged by intravascular injections (Fig. 4–23). In its winding course over the maxillary tuberosity it gives off one or two branches which, in company with the posterior alveolar nerves, enter the posterior superior alveolar canals (Figs. 4–6*A* and 4–20*B*). The artery continues along the outer surface of the bone to supply the buccal gingiva and mucous membrane in the molar and premolar region, with some of its branches reaching into the cheek. Occasionally the posterior superior alveolar artery arises from the buccal artery.

Arising separately or by a common trunk with the posterior superior alveolar, the infraorbital artery enters the inferior orbital fissure and accompanies the infraorbital nerve along the floor of the orbit. Emerging from the infraorbital foramen, it supplies the anterior part of the cheek and upper lip. In clinical practice, the artery rarely shows evidence of damage following an infraorbital block injection.

Pterygopalatine Ganglion and its Branches

The pterygopalatine ganglion with its branches, deeply placed within the fossa, has been characterized by Last[10] as "the ganglion of hay fever ('running nose and eyes'). It is a relay station between the superior salivatory nucleus in the pons and the lacrimal gland and mucous and serous glands of the palate, nose and paranasal sinuses." Its parasympathetic root is from the greater petrosal nerve, the sympathetic root from a plexus on the internal carotid artery via the deep petrosal nerve. These two groups of autonomic fibers unite in the foramen lacerum to reach the ganglion as the nerve of the pterygoid canal. The sensory root is from the maxillary nerve. The ganglion has orbital, nasal, pharyngeal and palatal branches of distribution. The two branches most often anesthetized by the dentist are the *nasopalatine nerve* and the *greater palatine nerve*. The former passes through the sphenopalatine foramen, crosses the roof of the nasal cavity and gains the nasal septum, which it follows in company with its contralateral fellow downward and forward to the incisive canal. The terminals supply the palatal gingival tissue in the incisor region (Fig. 4–12). A further communication is with the *greater palatine nerve* which reaches the palate after passing through the greater palatine canal (Fig. 4–27*C*). The anesthetist's approach to these nerves is described on page 48. *Lesser palatine nerves* also descend in the canal, but emerge at the lesser

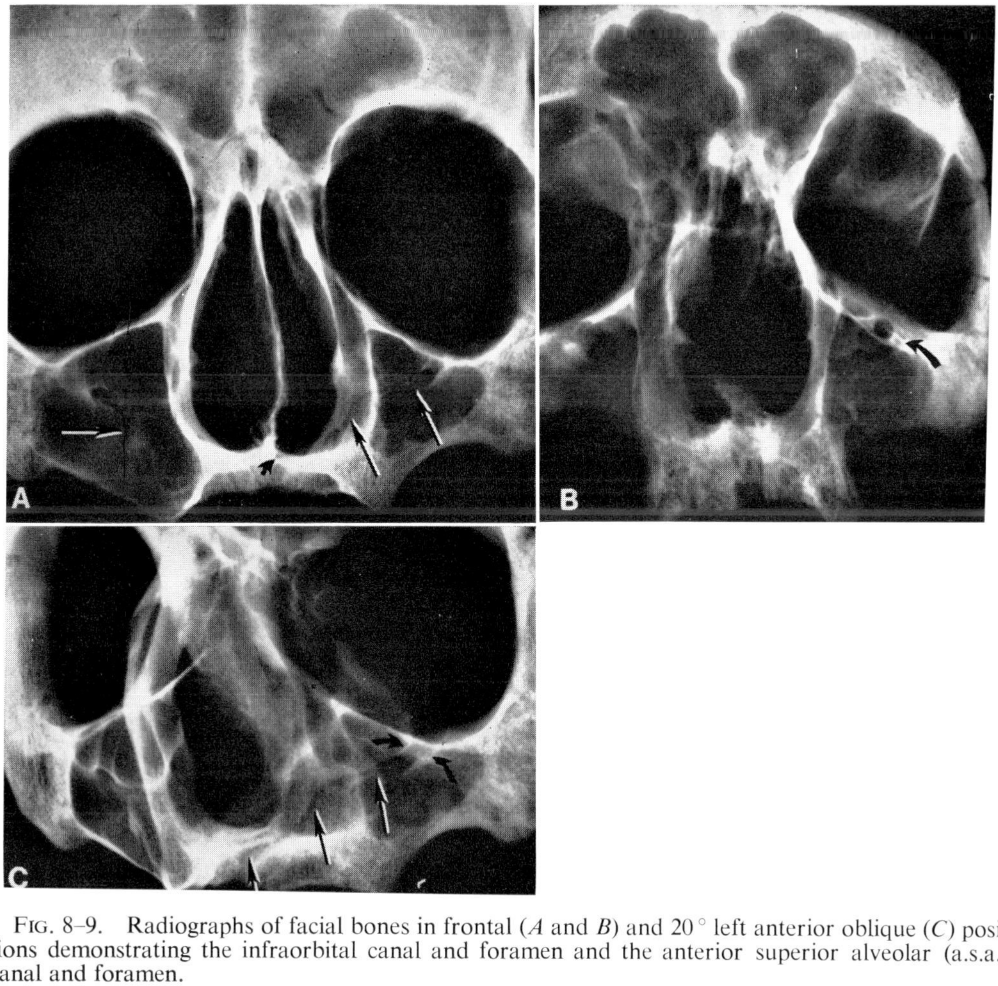

FIG. 8–9. Radiographs of facial bones in frontal (*A* and *B*) and 20° left anterior oblique (*C*) positions demonstrating the infraorbital canal and foramen and the anterior superior alveolar (a.s.a.) canal and foramen.

A: Hypoplastic left maxillary sinus with clearly defined a.s.a. canal, normal right sinus with only proximal portion of a.s.a. canal visible. Note anastomotic channels. In the midline a septal canal is visible to left of curved arrow. *B:* Anterior superior alveolar foramen lateral to and distinct from infraorbital foramen. *C:* Oblique view demonstrating the entirety of the a.s.a. vascular channel and infraorbital foramen and canal. (Courtesy of K. Dolan, M.D., Associate Professor of Radiology, University Hospital, Iowa City.)

palatine foramina and supply the soft palate and tonsil, so the anesthetist should by explanation prepare the patient for the sensory deficit which will occur after the injection of a local anesthetic into the canal.

Superior Alveolar Branches

The superior alveolar branches are usually described as posterior, middle and anterior superior alveolar nerves and vessels. Usually the *posterior superior alveolar nerves* are the most proximal maxillary nerves which the dentist anesthetizes. The nerve arises from the infraorbital nerve by one or more trunks which may divide into three or four branches before reaching the surface of the maxillary tuberosity, or on its surface, or after entering the foramina in the tuberosity (see Figs, 4–6*A*, 4–23 and 4–20*B*). In any case, one branch usually supplies the posterior gingival and adjacent buccal mucosal surfaces. In fact, the branch may at times replace the buccal nerve (p. 128). Branches of the posterior superior alveolar nerves to the teeth run within bony canals around the maxillary sinus in approximately the horizontal plane. The upper and smaller canal is at the level of the zygomatic process, and the lower is between this and the alveolar margin. These nerves also supply the mucosa of the maxillary sinus. The canal for the inferior branch of the posterior superior alveolar nerve may be traced as far anteriorly as the canine teeth. When the middle superior alveolar nerve is missing, these branches with those of the anterior superior alveolar nerve supply the first permanent molar. Anastomotic channels between the posterior and anterior superior alveolar neurovascular bundles are depicted in Figure 8–9*A*.

The *posterior superior alveolar* artery originates from the maxillary artery in the infratemporal fossa as the latter is entering the pterygopalatine fossa. It follows the tortuous path of the nerves to supply molar and premolar teeth and the adjacent periosteum, alveoli, gingiva and the mucosa of the maxillary sinus. As with the nerve, one branch does not enter a canal but runs beneath the zygomatic process to supply the buccinator muscle and oral mucosa.

The *middle superior alveolar nerves* and arteries supply the premolar teeth, or primary molars. Classic anatomical texts display no uniformity of description of such an arterial supply.[5,11] As for the corresponding nerves, a review of the literature concerning the distribution of the superior alveolar nerves as studied by the methods of dissection or anesthetic block technique[6] indicates that the middle superior alveolar nerves may often be missing, and that the superior alveolar nerve supply follows a pattern which may vary among individuals and bilaterally in a single person (Figs. 4–8 and 4–9). If the middle superior alveolar nerves and arteries are missing, presumably their function is supplied by the posterior and anterior superior alveolar branches.

The facial artery and vein in their previously described course cross the premolar root area (Figs. 4–17 and 8–2). The buccinator muscle from its bony attachment in the molar area passes forward in the cheek and, though its fibers may be pierced by the needle, it is seldom a consideration in the clinical anesthetization of teeth in the premolar areas (Figs. 8–3 and 8–5).

The fibers of the *anterior superior alveolar nerves* communicate between the infraorbital nerve and the tooth pulp. These fibers also supply some buccal alveolar bone and maxillary sinus mucous membrane. The anterior superior alveolar nerve is approximately one-third the size of the parent infraorbital nerve trunk, from which it originates rather far back in the infraorbital canal, sometimes posterior to the midpoint of the canal, and not uncommonly at the area of the tuberosity (Fig. 8–7). The anterior superior alveolar nerve runs forward from its origin on the lateral side of the parent trunk in a constant and large canal. The anterior superior alveolar nerve, at a point 7 or 8 mm lateral to the infraorbital foramen (Fig. 8–9*B*) and just below the zygomatico-maxillary suture, turns downward and then swings transversely across the anterior wall of the antrum to the lateral wall of the nasal chamber eventually ending at the anterior end of the inferior turbinate bone. It is between the medial aspect of the canine alveolus and the narial margin that the nerve "gives off its first conspicuous dental branch to the canine, and smaller branches may be traced to the incisors."[9]

Jones,[9] in his classic descriptive paper, draws one's attention to the fact that in surgery of the maxillary sinus it is important to remember that the canal is large and constant, as a corrective to the common impression that the anterior superior alveolar nerve consists of small branches running in small bony canals down the anterior wall of the sinus. Also of importance is the real contribution these nerves and accompanying vessels make to the septal and lateral walls of the nasal cavity.

Obviously, the anterior superior alveolar nerve at times may be anesthetized by supraperiosteal infiltration, infraorbital or posterior superior alveolar (tuberosity) blocks, and always by second division blocks. These blocks and their relative anatomical landmarks have been described in Chapter 4.

The *anterior superior alveolar artery* branches from the infraorbital artery and follows the course of the companion nerves to anastomose with branches of the posterior superior alveolar artery (Fig. 8–9*A*) and near the piriform aperture with the nasal arteries. The infraorbital artery ends on the face, with a distribution similar to the terminals of the infraorbital nerves and forming anastomotic connections with the angular, superior labial branches of the facial, the nasal and lacrimal branches of the ophthalmic and the transverse facial arteries.

Infraorbital Branches

Infraorbital branches from the maxillary nerve and artery are obviously relatively and frequently concerned with local anesthesia. The gingiva overlying the central incisors and the pulp nerves contains the terminal receptors for sensations eventually reaching the central nervous system via the maxillary nerve (Fig. 4–10). Immediately beneath the gingiva lies the exquisitely sensitive periosteum which covers the bone over the tooth root. In this area the most anterior and terminal branches of the infraorbital nerve supply the lower eyelid, the skin of the nose, the mucous membrane of the mouth and the skin of the lip (Fig. 4–17). The gingival branches, with those of the anterior superior alveolar nerves, contribute to a rich network of nervous and vascular tissues which responds pronouncedly to noxious stimuli.

The network of nerve fibers, extending between the central incisor and canine teeth and accompanied by blood and lymph vessels, runs in neurovascular bundles which pass from the gingiva via perforations in the alveolar bone and via the infraorbital foramen to the parent trunk.

MANDIBULAR NERVE

The mandibular nerve was briefly described (page 122). In its short course of 2 to 3 mm the *trunk* provides a branch to innervate the meninges and the medial pterygoid muscle. It then divides into an anterior and a posterior division.

Buccal Nerve

The *anterior division* of the mandibular nerve is mainly muscular, with one sensory branch, the buccal nerve. The muscular branches are to the temporalis, lateral pterygoid, and masseter muscles. The sensory buccal nerve supplies the mucosa of the inner surface of the cheek and adjacent gingiva and communicates with branches of the facial nerve. Generally it emerges between the two heads of the lateral pterygoid muscle (Fig. 8–5*c*) and runs downward and forward close to, or in a fascial tunnel attached to, the medial side of the deep tendon of the temporalis muscle or sometimes within the substance of the muscle near its anterior border. After emerging at the anterior border of the superficial and deep temporal tendons, the nerve reaches the buccinator muscle (Figs. 8–3 and 8–5*d*) where it breaks up into branches. Single branches of the nerve penetrate the buccinator muscle and innervate almost all the mucosa of the cheek, except a posterior superior area which may receive fibers from the gingival branch of the posterior superior alveolar nerve. The buccal nerve is in reciprocal relationship to the posterior superior alveolar nerve (page 126) and thus either one may innervate a larger or smaller area. The dentist is often concerned with the buccal nerve distribution to the buccal gingiva of the mandibular second premolar and first premolar. The area may be enlarged to include all teeth distal to the canine, or the nerve may be excluded from supplying any part of the gingiva.

The *posterior division* of the mandibular nerve is largely sensory; only the mylohyoid nerve is muscular. The auriculotemporal nerve is first given off; then, a little lower and medial to the lateral pterygoid muscle, the posterior division gives rise to the lingual and inferior alveolar branches. The lingual and inferior alveolar branches soon arise as the two largest branches from the mandibular nerve (Figs. 4–31 and 8–6). They continue downward to lie in the outer surface of the medial pterygoid muscle, where they are at first between the medial and lateral pterygoid muscle and then between the medial pterygoid muscle and ramus of the mandible (Fig. 8–5*b*).

Auriculotemporal Nerve

The auriculotemporal nerve passes backward, lying medial to the neck of the mandible and above the maxillary vessels (Fig. 8–5*a*). It provides part of the innervation to the joint, ear, temple and parotid gland. It also conveys to the parotid gland the postganglionic secretomotor fibers from the otic ganglion.

Lingual Nerve

The large lingual nerve follows a course downward, forward and medial to the inferior alveolar nerve (Figs. 4–31 and 4–34), separated from it by the interpterygoid fascia (Figs. 4–35 and 8–3). The two nerves may communicate. Near its origin the lingual nerve is joined by the chorda tympani nerve (Figs. 4–31, 4–35, and 8–6), which subserves the sensation of taste in the anterior two-thirds of the tongue and carries the parasympathetic secretomotor fibers to the submandibular and sublingual glands. As it leaves the masticator space to enter the mouth, the lingual nerve is in a superficial position, subject to injury from a needle point or the blade of a scalpel injudiciously directed lingual to the retromolar pad. The lingual nerve enters the oral cavity about 1 mm below and behind the third molar. It is superficial enough that the index finger may be used to press the nerve against the bone of the mandible; the resulting sensation is unpleasant. At this point the nerve lies beneath the mandibular origin of the superior constrictor muscle, at the lower end of the pterygomandibular raphe. Here, at the upper end of the mylohyoid line, the nerve turns sharply forward on the superior medial surface of the mylohyoid muscle to continue into the oral cavity (Fig. 8–5*c*). In the connective tissue-filled niche between the mylohyoid and hyoglossus muscles the lingual nerve suspends the submandibular ganglion, curves under the submandibular duct from lateral to medial, and then distributes to the mucous membrane of the anterior two-thirds of the tongue.

Inferior Alveolar and Mylohyoid Nerves

The inferior alveolar nerve beneath the lateral pterygoid muscle swings sharply downward and laterally, to enter the mandibular foramen between the sphenomandibular ligament and the ramus. Sicher and Dubrul[12] emphasize that the nerve has no contact with the mandible above the entrance into the mandibular canal. However, Hollinshead[7] suggests that the nerves are in contact with the mandible for a very short distance above the spine of the lingula. Some oral surgeons performing neurectomies from an anterior intraoral approach report that in these cases the nerve may approximate the mandible. The nerve lies anterior to its vessels and behind and lateral to the lingual nerve (Figs. 4–34, 4–35 and 8–3). Before entering the mandibular foramen the inferior alveolar nerve releases the mylohyoid nerve which pierces the sphenomandibular ligament (Figs. 4–34 and 4–35) and in company with its vessels runs in the mylohyoid groove of the mandible (Figs. 4–31 and 8–5*b*) and, passing externally to the mylohyoid muscle, supplies it and the anterior belly of the digastric muscle with motor fibers.

The nerve has sensory fibers and the cutaneous branch, when present, supplies the skin on the inferior and anterior side of the mental protuberance. "In about 10 per cent of the examined cadavers, a twig of the terminal sensory branch of the mylohyoid nerve enters the mandible in the mental region and may participate in the nerve supply to the lower incisor."[12] The inferior alveolar nerve in the mandibular canal runs forward to the premolar area where the cutaneous mental nerve arises, innervating the skin of the chin, the skin and mucous membrane of the lip and the facial alveolar surface. The continuation of the inferior alveolar nerve is called the *incisive branch* and supplies the canine and incisor teeth and adjacent facial gingiva.

THE SUPERIOR AND INFERIOR DENTAL PLEXUS

In the bony alveolar canals of the maxillae there is a mingling of the fibers from all the superior alveolar nerves to form a superior dental plexus. From this plexus arise the terminal superior dental branches, supplying the maxillary teeth, the superior gingival branches, supplying the gingivae, and sensory branches to the mucosa of the maxillary sinus.

In the mandible the inferior alveolar nerve divides into a variable number of branches enumerated as posterior, middle and anterior sets.[12] These nerves, with their corresponding arteries and veins, give rise to an inferior alveolar or dental plexus which innervates the mandibular teeth and periodontium. Where the gingiva is not supplied by the buccal nerve, perforating interdental nerves from the plexus provide the innervation.

Branches from the superior or inferior dental nerve enter the apical foramen of each tooth where they unite to form a common pulpal nerve.[3] In an earlier study[4] of 200 sectioned noncarious human teeth, it was observed that the nerve bundle accompanies the blood vessels in the long axis of the root, and breaks up into 3 or 4 main longitudinal fiber bundles when reaching the crown portion of the tooth. These bundles pass peripherally to supply all wall surfaces of the tooth.

The innervation of the periodontal membrane and the gingival tissues was reviewed by Anderson, Hannam and Matthews.[1] In summary, the periodontal ligament contains nerve fibers that run from the apical region of the root toward the gingival margin, joined by fibers that enter the ligament laterally through foramina in the alveolar bone. These fibers are from the superior or inferior dental nerves. The gingival tissues are innervated by terminal branches of the periodontal fibers as well as by fibers from the infraorbital and palatine or lingual, mental and buccal nerves as appropriate. Still, Ten Cate writes, "It is surprising how little is known concerning the innervation of the periodontium, when its important functional role is considered . . . as with the development of the vascular supply, a hiatus exists in our knowledge between early developmental stages and the mature ligament with respect to innervation."[13]

LYMPH DRAINAGE

Except to mention a few classically described and particularly pertinent lymph nodes, the lymphatic drainage will not be discussed. One might also consider the possible effect of lymphatic flow in aiding the spread of the local anesthetic solution, for instance in the case of the infraorbital or mental nerve blocks.

The lymph flow of the face drains into three groups of nodes: (1) the *submental* nodes draining the chin and tongue tip; (2) the *submandibular* nodes draining the central forehead and frontal sinuses through the anterior half of the nose and maxillary sinus to the upper lip and lower part of the face, including the side of the tongue and the floor of the mouth; and (3) the *preauricular* group of nodes draining the remaining portion of the forehead, temple, the orbital contents and the cheek. Among the deep nodes the *retropharyngeal* nodes are particularly concerned with the drainage of the nasal fossae and the paranasal sinuses, the hard and soft palate, the nasopharynx and oropharynx.

The interested reader and student should consult an authoritative treatment of lymphatic drainage, and might well start with the references in the anatomy texts contained in the Bibliography for this chapter.

BIBLIOGRAPHY

1. Anderson, D. J., Hannam, A. G. and Matthews, B.: Sensory mechanisms in mammalian teeth and their supporting structures. Physiol. Rev. *50*:171, 1970.
2. Bassett, D. L.: *A Stereoscopic Atlas of Human Anatomy*, Section II, Head and Neck. Baltimore, Williams and Wilkins Co., 1954.
3. Bernick, Sol: Innervation of teeth and periodontium after enzymatic removal of collagenous elements. Oral Surg., Oral Med., Oral Path. *10*:323, 1957.
4. Bernick, Sol: Innervation of the human tooth. Anat. Rec. *101*:81, 1948.
5. Romanes, G. J., ed.: *Cunningham's Textbook of Anatomy*, 13th ed. London, Oxford University Press, 1968.
6. Hayden, Jess, Jr.: The innervation of the maxillary first permanent and primary molars as determined by deposition of local anesthetic solutions. Acta Odont. Scand. *23*:147, 1965.
7. Hollinshead, W. H.: *Anatomy for Surgeons*, 2nd ed., 3 Vols. Vol. I, The Head and Neck. New York, Hoeber, Inc., 1968.
8. Humphrey, Tryphena: Reflex activity in the oral and facial area of the human fetus. In *Oral Sensation and Perception* (Bosma, J. F., ed.). Springfield, Charles C Thomas, 1970.
9. Jones, F. W.: The anterior superior alveolar nerve and vessels. J. Anat. *73*:588, 1939.
10. Last, R. J.: *Anatomy, Regional and Applied*, 4th ed. Boston, Little, Brown, 1966.
11. Anson, B. J., ed.: *Morris' Human Anatomy*, 12th ed. New York, McGraw-Hill, 1966.
12. Sicher, Harry and Dubrul, E. L.: *Oral Anatomy*, 5th ed. St. Louis, C. V. Mosby Co., 1970.
13. Ten Cate, A. R.: Development of the periodontium. In *Biology of the Periodontium* (Melcher, A. H. and Bowen, W. H., eds.). New York, Academic Press, 1969.
14. Woodburne, R. T.: *Essentials of Human Anatomy*, 4th ed. New York, Oxford University Press, 1969.
15. Worth, H. M.: *Principles and Practice of Oral Radiologic Interpretation*. Chicago, Yearbook Medical Publishers, 1963, p. 212.

Atlases of Sectional Anatomy

16. Eycleshymer, A. C. and Shoemaker, D. M.: *A Cross-section Anatomy*. New York, Appleton-Century-Crofts, 1970.
17. Kampmeier, O. F., Cooper, A. R. and Jones, T. S.: *A Frontal Section Anatomy of the Head and Neck*. Urbana, University of Illinois Press, 1957.
18. Truex, R. C. and Kellner, C. E.: *Detailed Atlas of Head and Neck*. New York, Oxford University Press, 1948.

Chapter

9

Local Anesthetics

C. L. Mitchell, Ph.D.

Local anesthetics are undoubtedly the most frequently used drugs in the practice of dentistry. A thorough understanding of these agents is, therefore, important to insure their rational clinical use.

As employed in dentistry, local anesthetics are drugs which reversibly block nerve conduction when applied locally to nerve tissue in appropriate concentrations. This definition contains several points important to remember: (1) reversibility of the blocking action, (2) application to nerve tissue and (3) necessity for an appropriate concentration. Obviously, if an agent (*e.g.*, ethanol) blocks nerve conduction in an irreversible manner, it is not useful as a local anesthetic. Second, local anesthetics must reach the nerve tissue in order to be active. Moreover, they must reach it in an appropriate concentration or they will not block nerve conduction.

There are many local anesthetic agents available. When there are many agents for a particular use this generally implies that none of them is very good. This is not true for local anesthetics. Many of them are quite good. None of them fulfills the criteria set forth for the "ideal" agent (Table 1). However, some of these criteria are self-contradictory. For example, potency and toxicity go hand in hand; the more potent an agent, the greater its toxicity. Again, the more rapid the onset, the shorter the duration. The more water soluble, the less fat soluble—yet fat solubility is essential for penetration of tissues.

Our present understanding of how local anesthetics block nerve conduction and of why some criteria for the ideal agent are contradictory will be discussed. Moreover, since these drugs produce effects on other organs as well as their desired local anesthetic effect, we must consider their toxicity. Finally, since there are various agents from which to choose, the similarities and differences among agents will be examined.

TABLE 1. Criteria for an Ideal Local Anesthetic

Should be potent
Should be nontoxic (both to nerve tissue and to the whole body)
Should have a rapid onset
Should have a long duration
Should be water soluble
Should be stable in solution
Should be free from allergic or idiosyncratic reactions
Should be sterilizable without deterioration
Should have an action which is reversible

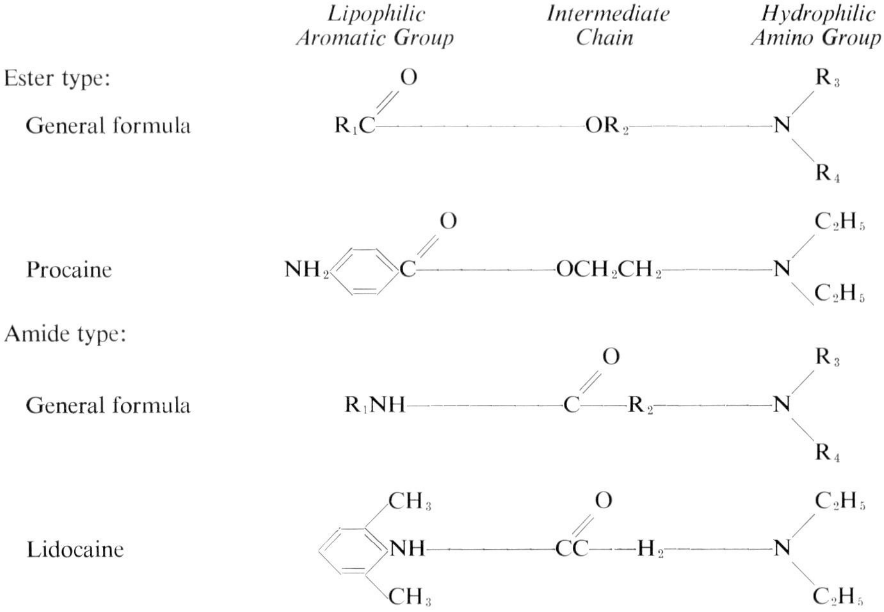

FIG. 9–1. Structural formulae of local anesthetics.

CHEMISTRY

The first local anesthetic known was cocaine, introduced as a topical anesthetic in 1884. It was not until 1904, with the introduction of procaine, that a safe local anesthetic drug was available for injection purposes. Although cocaine is a natural substance, all the agents in current use in dentistry are synthetic products.

Local anesthetics are weakly basic amines, with a pKa in the range of 7 to 9 and poorly soluble in water. They form salts with strong acids and most often are supplied for clinical use as the hydrochloride salt. These salts are freely soluble in water. The resulting solution is acidic (pH 6 or less).

The agents in current use have three parts to the molecule (Fig 9–1): (1) a lipophilic aromatic group, (2) an intermediate chain, (3) a hydrophilic amino group.

Changes in any part of the molecule may change the potency or toxicity of the drug. For example, an increase in the length of the intermediate chain leads to an increase in potency and toxicity.

Local anesthetics may be classed into two major types of amines (Fig. 9–1): (1) those which contain an ester linkage, and (2) those which contain an amide linkage. This difference in chemistry results in significant differences in pharmacology, particularly in relation to metabolism and toxicity.

GENERAL PHARMACOLOGY

Absorption

Local anesthetics vary considerably in their ability to penetrate tissue. This difference can be explained on the basis of the pKa of the compound. Recall that local anesthetics are bases which readily form acid salts; moreover, the salt form is usually employed in clinical practice. In solution, local anesthetics always occur in two forms: the ionized and nonionized forms. This can best be illustrated by the standard equations for the behavior of a base and its salts (Fig. 9–2).

The concentration of the ionized and non-

$$BHCl \xrightarrow{H_2O} \underset{\text{ionized form}}{BH^+} + Cl^+$$

$$BH^+ + H_2O \rightleftharpoons \underset{\text{free base}}{B} + H_3O^+$$

FIG. 9–2. Equations for the behavior of a base and its hydrochloride salt in water.

ionized form in any solution is dependent upon the ionization constant (pKa) of the compound and the pH of the solution (see Table 2). The higher the pKa of a compound, the less free base will exist at the same pH level. The importance of this information is the fact that only the free base can readily penetrate tissue membranes. The higher the pKa of the compound, the less free base will be available at physiological pH (7.4). For example, at pH 7.4 approximately 20 per cent of lidocaine hydrochloride is in the free base form whereas only 2 per cent of procaine hydrochloride is in free base form.

The injectable solution of local anesthetics is acidic. The actual pH varies with the agent and the vasoconstrictor present. In any case, the pH will usually be less than 6. As can be seen from Table 2, there is little free base available at a pH of 6 or less. Fortunately, the buffering effect of the tissue fluids leads to an increase in the pH and the consequent release of the free base (Fig. 9–3). However, this does not occur instantly. The lower the pH of the solution, the larger the volume of injection and the higher the concentration of the vasoconstrictor present in the solution, the longer it will take for the tissue to neutralize the injected solution. For example, after the injection of 1 ml of 2 per cent lidocaine or procaine hydrochloride solution at pH 3, the pH of the tissue may not return to normal until after 45 minutes.[1] The significance of this point is the delay in action of the local anesthetic, since a sufficient quantity of the free base must be liberated before anesthesia can occur. It should also be mentioned that products produced by the microorganisms present in infected tissue tend to lower extracellular pH. This diminishes the buffering capacity of the tissue and thus reduces the amount of free base liberated. Consequently, the effectiveness of the local anesthetic will be reduced when injected into infected areas.

TABLE 2. Per Cent Distribution of Ionized and Nonionized Forms of Procaine and Lidocaine at Different pH

	Procaine (pKa 8.93)		*Lidocaine (pKa 7.85)*	
pH	*Ionized* %	*Nonionized* %	*Ionized* %	*Nonionized* %
6	99.9	0.09	99	1
7	99.1	0.9	90	10
7.4	98.0	2.0	80	20
8	91.1	7.9	50	50

It should also be pointed out, however, that the presence or absence of anesthesia depends on the concentration of the anesthetic in contact with the nerve fibers rather than on the concentration in the surrounding tissue. In other words, when the local anesthetic is properly placed less anesthetic is required than when the injection is poorly placed. This is true regardless of the pKa of the compound.

Mechanism of Action

The sequence of changes in a nerve fiber following the application of a local anesthetic agent can best be described by following the electrophysiological changes. The first effect seen is an increase in the threshold for electrical stimulation. This is followed, in sequence, by a reduction in the size of the action potential, a slowing of the conduction velocity, and finally the cessation of impulse propagation altogether (provided the concentration of the local anesthetic is sufficient to produce blockade). Although the precise mechanism whereby local anesthetics produce their effect is not known, it is possible to explain, at least partially, the action of local anesthetics in relation to the ionic theory of nervous activity.

The resting single nerve fiber has a polarized membrane, positively charged on the outside and negatively charged on the inside. This resting membrane potential is caused by a difference in the ion concentrations

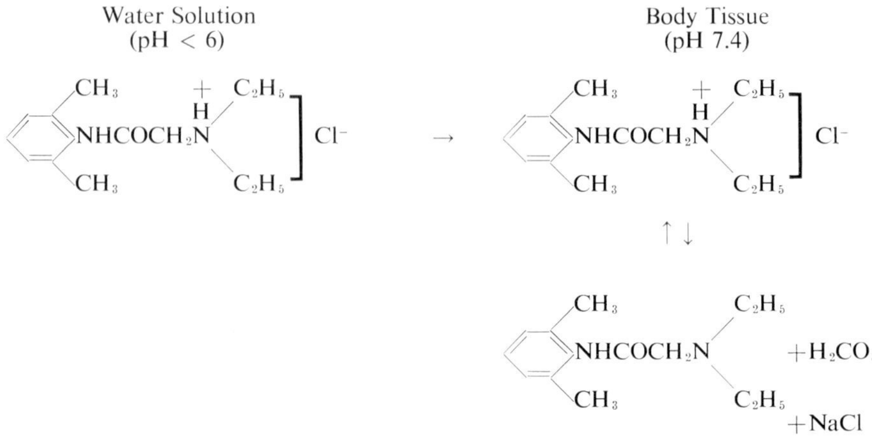

FIG. 9–3. Lidocaine injected as the hydrochloride salt is buffered by the extracellular fluid and the free base is liberated.

across the membrane. For example, the concentration of sodium ions is larger outside than inside; the reverse is true for potassium ions.

The fundamental process in nerve conduction is a large transient increase in the permeability of the membrane to sodium. Local anesthetics block conduction by interfering with this increase in sodium permeability.[2] The precise mechanism is not known, since the mechanism whereby the sodium permeability increases when a nerve is stimulated is not entirely known. In the nerve at rest there is evidence that calcium ions are involved in blocking the passage of sodium ions through the membrane. Stimulation of the fiber may remove the calcium ions or change their orientation with the result that sodium can penetrate the membrane.[3,4] It has been postulated that the local anesthetics act in a manner similar to calcium.[5] It has also been suggested that local anesthetics act by closing the pores through which ions move,[6] or affect permeability by increasing the degree of disorder of the membrane.[7]

It has been mentioned that the free base is necessary to penetrate tissue. There has been a difference of opinion, however, as to whether the free base or the cation is the active form once the local anesthetic has penetrated the nerve. The most recent evidence suggests that either form may be active but that the cation probably plays the major role.[8,9]

Whatever the mechanism by which local anesthetics act and whatever the active form, from the practical point of view it is important to remember that they will block conduction only if the concentration is high enough. Otherwise only an increase in threshold, a reduction in the size of the action potential and a slowing of the conduction velocity are obtained. This means that, if the initiating stimulus is of sufficient intensity to overcome the elevation in threshold, the fiber will conduct and the result may be the presence of pain.

It is known, however, that different concentrations of anesthetic are required to block conduction in fibers of different sizes. As a general rule, small nerve fibers are more susceptible to the action of local anesthetics than are large fibers. Some overlap occurs, nevertheless. For example, it has been shown that some A delta fibers are blocked with lower concentrations of anesthetic than are most of the C fibers[10] (which are smaller than the A delta fibers). Clinically, the general order of loss of function is as follows: (1) pain, (2) temperature, (3) touch, (4) proprioception, and (5) skeletal muscle tone. Since this order is indicative of the sensitivity of these fibers to local anesthetics, it is not surprising that the return of function will occur in the reverse order.

Toxicity

In addition to blocking conduction in nerve trunks, local anesthetics interfere with the function of all excitable tissue. Thus, they have important effects on the central nervous system and all forms of muscle fibers. Clinically, the toxicity of these agents is manifested by effects on the central nervous system and the cardiovascular system, and is due to their absorption systemically.

Toxicity of the Central Nervous System

With respect to the central nervous system (CNS), all of the local anesthetics will cause stimulation. This may vary from mild restlessness to severe convulsions. In general, the more potent the anesthetic, the more readily convulsions may be produced. Excessive stimulation, regardless of the cause, is followed by depression, and death may occur due to respiratory failure. If excessive stimulation occurs it can be suppressed by the intravenous injection of an ultrashort-acting barbiturate such as methohexital (Brevital). This procedure is not without its hazards, however, since barbiturates, being respiratory depressants, may enhance any subsequent respiratory depressant effect from the local anesthetic.

It has been suggested that the stimulation seen with local anesthetics is, in fact, due solely to a depression of neuronal activity.[11] The apparent stimulation is perhaps due to a selective depression of inhibitory neurons (*i.e.*, they are more sensitive and thus a smaller concentration of local anesthetic will block them).

Occasionally, with the amide derivatives and in particular lidocaine, gross signs of CNS depression may be seen before or instead of convulsions. They are manifested by signs of drowsiness and depressed respiration. Also, with any of the agents, it is possible to get a localized anesthesia in the pons following fifth-nerve block. If the injection is made with a very fine needle, some of the anesthetic may be deposited in the subperineural space of the nerve and a small volume of solution may reach the subarachnoid space. When this occurs, apnea and/or hypotension occur rapidly. Since respiratory depression is the most frequent cause of death from local anesthetic toxicity, one must always be prepared to administer artificial respiration.

Toxicity of the Cardiovascular System

All local anesthetics used in dentistry have profound effects on the cardiovascular system. They: (1) increase the refractory period of the heart, (2) slow conduction of electrical impulses within the heart, (3) decrease the contractile force of the heart, (4) produce vasodilatation, probably by a direct effect on smooth muscle. In other words, they lower blood pressure by weakening the heart and causing vasodilatation.

These effects may occur independently of effects on the central nervous system or in conjunction with them. As with the CNS effects, potency of the local anesthetic and toxicity to the cardiovascular system go hand in hand.

Allergic Reactions

Hypersensitivity to local anesthetics is manifested as allergic dermatitis, asthma or the anaphylactic reaction. The allergic state is most readily induced by topical applications over a period of time, but may be produced by even a single injection. Contact dermatitis may also occur, but usually develops only after prolonged exposure. This is clearly a hazard to the dentist, however, since small amounts may routinely be spilled on the hands.

Metabolism

A local anesthetic (or any other drug) will act until the concentration is low enough that it is no longer sufficient to produce the desired effect. In the case of local anesthetics, this occurs by their being picked up by the bloodstream, from which they are redistributed to other tissue, metabolized and excreted.

The two major chemical groups, the esters and the amides, are metabolized in different ways. The ester type of agents are hydrolyzed by the plasma cholinesterase, also known as procaine esterase, and by esterases in the liver. They are hydrolyzed to their component acids and alcohols; for example, procaine is hydrolyzed to p-aminobenzoic acid and diethylaminoethanol. Metabolic degradation by plasma esterase is an important route for esters. The rate of hydrolysis in plasma varies with the compounds, being very rapid for piperocaine (Metycaine) and absent for dibucaine (Nupercaine). The other ester-type agents fall between these two extremes. As might be expected, the duration of action of these agents correlates well with their affinity for plasma cholinesterase.

In contrast to the esters, the amides are metabolized only in the endoplasmic reticulum of the liver. As with the esters, however, the rate of metabolic degradation varies considerably among agents and accounts, at least in part, for the differences in duration of action.

USE OF VASOCONSTRICTORS

Sympathomimetic amines are widely used with local anesthetics. When injected with a local anesthetic, they cause local vasoconstriction which slows the absorption of the local anesthetic.

This slowing of absorption: (1) prolongs the duration of action, (2) decreases the amount of local anesthetic needed, and (3) reduces the danger of systemic toxicity.

For a given dose of local anesthetic, the higher the concentration of sympathomimetic amine present, the longer the duration of the local anesthesia. However, this increase in duration is obtained only at a price. The greater the concentration of sympathomimetic amine, the greater the chance of: (1) tissue damage due to ischemia, or (2) systemic toxicity to the sympathomimetic amine.

The most commonly used agent is epinephrine. It has been used in concentrations of from 1:100,000 to 1:20,000.

Patients with hyperthyroidism, hypertension and heart disease are particularly susceptible to the pressor and cardiac effects of epinephrine. Also, it is well to remember that patients with long-standing respiratory disease (*e.g.*, asthma and emphysema) usually have accompanying heart disease. Therefore, epinephrine or other vasoconstrictors must be used with caution, if at all, in these patients.

PHARMACOLOGY OF SPECIFIC AGENTS

Many local anesthetic agents are available. Some are effective both topically and by injection. Some are effective only if injected; some are used only topically because they are extremely toxic when injected. The list which follows consists of only the more commonly used agents in dentistry. It is better to learn to use one or two of these agents well than to use many agents poorly.

Esters

Procaine (Novocain) was the first synthetic local anesthetic. It is relatively less potent and less toxic than the other agents which will be mentioned. It has a rapid onset but a short duration of action. As with other agents, its duration of action will depend somewhat on the concentration of vasoconstrictor present. In dentistry, it is used as a 2 per cent solution of procaine hydrochloride.

Propoxycaine (Ravocaine) is more potent and more toxic than procaine. Also, it does not penetrate tissues as well as procaine. In dentistry, it is used as a 0.4 per cent solution with 2 per cent procaine. This combination produces a rapid onset and fairly long duration of anesthesia.

Amides

Lidocaine (Xylocaine) has a fairly rapid onset and long duration of action. It is 2 to 3 times as potent (and toxic) as procaine. It is effective when used without a vasoconstrictor but the rate of absorption and toxicity are increased and the duration of action shortened. It appears to be the agent of choice for individuals with whom a vasoconstrictor should not be used. In dentistry it is used in a 2 per cent concentration and has become the standard by which other agents are compared.

Mepivacaine (Carbocaine) has pharmacological properties quite similar to those of lidocaine. Its action is said to be more rapid in onset and more prolonged than that of lidocaine.

Prilocaine (Citanest) also has pharmacological properties similar to lidocaine. Its action, however, is slower in onset and more prolonged than that of lidocaine. A unique toxic effect of high doses is methemoglobinemia, which can be treated by methylene blue.

BIBLIOGRAPHY

1. Björn, H.: The neutralization of acid local anesthetic solutions in the tissues. Svensk Tandläk. T. *40*:853, 1947.
2. Taylor, R. E.: Effect of procaine on electrical properties of squid axon membrane. Amer. J. Physiol. *196*:1071, 1959.
3. Hashimura, S. and Wright, E. B.: Effect of ionic environment on excitability and electrical properties of frog single nerve fiber. J. Neurophysiol. *21*:34, 1958.
4. Mueller, P.: On the kinetics of potential, electromotance, and chemical change in the excitable system of nerve. J. Gen. Physiol. *42*:193, 1958.
5. Blaustein, M. P. and Goldman, D. E.: Competitive action of calcium and procaine on lobster axon. J. Gen. Physiol. *49*:1043, 1966.
6. Shanes, A. M.: Drugs and nerve conduction. Ann. Rev. Pharmacol. *3*:185, 1963.
7. Metcalfe, J. C. and Burgen, A. S. V.: Relaxation of anaesthetics in the presence of cytomembranes. Nature *220*:587, 1968.
8. Ritchie, J. M. and Ritchie, B. R.: Local anesthetics: Effect of pH on activity. Science *162*:1394, 1968.
9. Narahashi, T. and Frazier, D. T.: Site of action and active form of local anesthetics in nerve fibers. Fed. Proc. *27*:1092, 1968.
10. Nathan, P. W. and Sears, T. A.: Some factors concerned in differential nerve block by local anaesthetics. J. Physiol. *157*:565, 1961.
11. Frank, G. B. and Sanders, H. D.: A proposed common mechanism of action for general and local anesthetics in the central nervous system. Brit. J. Pharmacol. *21*:1, 1963.

Section IV

History

Chapter 10

A Survey of Anesthesia, Sedation and Analgesia as Related to Dentistry

SURGERY WITHOUT ANESTHESIA

If we look back to the early 1800s, there were no anesthetics as we know them today, and unfortunately individuals who required surgery were faced with the choice of dying "whole" or electing the slender hope of surviving the shock produced by surgery without anesthesia. A case in point is that of a lad with a pea-like mass, originating on a carious tooth, that had grown to envelop almost the whole of his mouth. The 14-year-old patient, Jesse Lay, was nearing the point of suffocation which forced him to undergo mandibular hemisection without anesthesia.[11] It is a well-documented fact that this was not an isolated occurrence in the days before general anesthetics.[22]

As far as Jesse Lay was concerned, in 1810 the drugs available for analgesia were alcohol, opium, henbane (hyoscamos), cocaine, and mandragora (mandrake). The ancients utilized hypnotic and narcotic effects centuries before Christ,[5] but today such methods are not suitable for anesthesia. Not until 1806 was the active ingredient of opium derived by Sertunius, who eventually named it "morphine" after Morpheus, the Roman god of sleep. At this time only opium and alcohol had value in the control of pain in surgery; when taken in doses sufficient to cause sleep, their effect was always respiratory depression, often resulting in death, and postoperative nausea was frequent. Because of this the use of these drugs was discontinued. It was not until 1855 that opium was first administered with a syringe by the Scottish physician Alexander Wood. The clinical use of cocaine, obtained from coca leaves and long known in South America, was delayed almost another 30 years.

NITROUS OXIDE

Practical inhalation anesthesia was discovered in 1844 by Horace Wells. According to Archer, "Horace Wells was a sensitive and compassionate young dental surgeon as has been indicated in his letters. The sufferings he caused when he extracted teeth troubled

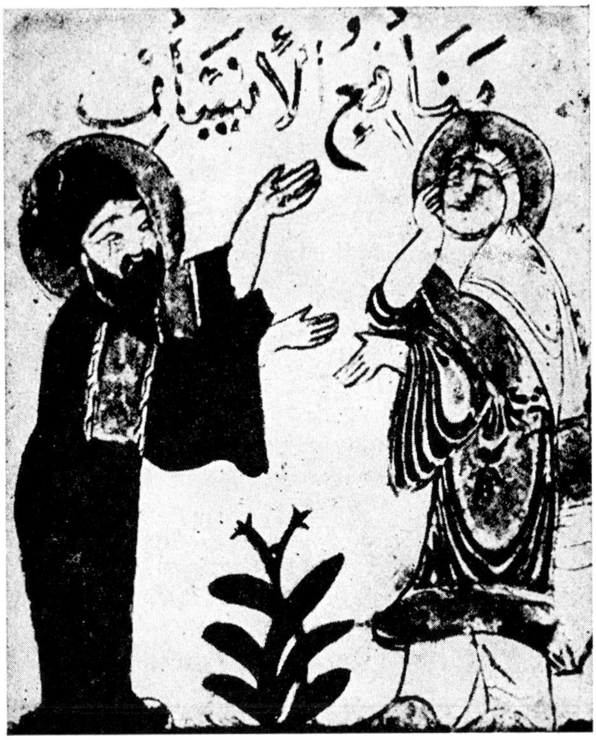

FIG. 10–1. The dentist examines a patient. In many of the medical manuscripts of the Middle Ages, miniatures which are often true works of art are found depicting medical and surgical treatment. The leaf shown from an Arabic manuscript of the thirteenth century displays a dental theme. From the right, a patient appears with her hand held to her swollen cheek; she is received by a dentist of very Oriental appearance. Above the heads of the two is written in Arabic, "It is the blessing of the teeth!" Between the figures, at the foot of the picture, is a medicinal herb. It is not accidental that the drawing does not show a tooth extraction, since the Arab view of dental treatment was quite conservative and emphasized the treatment of tooth disease with a highly developed stock of medicinals. Among the most advanced Arab authors of the time who discussed dental problems were Abukasim, Avicenna and Razes. (Pindborg, J. J. and Marvitz, L.: *The Dentist in Art.* Courtesy of Quadrangle Books, Inc.)

him greatly. Because the extraction of teeth was one of the most frequently performed dental operations, his mind was constantly occupied with the thought of discovering some way to prevent the terrible pain which accompanied the operation."[1] In December of 1844 Wells attended a meeting called by Professor Colton, a chemist, who desired to demonstrate for entertainment and fun the effect of nitrous oxide gas. (For example, those who inhaled the gas often broke into uncontrolled laughter.) Wells inhaled some of the gas and as a result his wife said "he made a spectacle of himself."

Perhaps Wells, a profound student, was analyzing his own reactions as he watched Mr. Samuel Cooley severely "bark his shins" and exhibit no pain. One decisive thought crystallized—surgery without pain.

Wells immediately sought out a former student, John Riggs, to discuss the benefits and risks of making a man "dead drunk" by means of nitrous oxide gas. Arriving at a reasoned conclusion, they courageously proved it the next morning. On October 11, 1844, Riggs extracted a tooth from the anesthetized Wells. Later Riggs wrote: "We knew not whether death or success confronted us. It was *terra incognito* we were bound to explore—The result is known to the world; no one but Wells and myself knew to what point the inhalation was to be carried. The result was painfully problematical to us but the great law of nature, hitherto unknown, was kind to us and a grand discovery was born into the world."[1]

Wells devoted the next months to experiments which, presumably in January 1845, led to the demonstration of nitrous oxide anesthesia[1] for the extraction of a tooth before the senior medical students of John C. Warren at Harvard University. The demonstration was a failure. The patient moaned and the gathering laughed and dispersed. However, the patient asserted that he had felt no pain.

Nitrous oxide inhalation for *sedation* was described in a 1908 textbook based on a series of lectures on general anesthetics in dentistry delivered by W. H. DeFord,[12] who was a professor of dentistry at the University of Iowa and later Dean of the College of Dentistry at Drake University. DeFord relates that during the fourth annual dental alumni clinic at the University of Iowa (Feb. 4, 1907) there was a successful clinical demonstration of the sedative effects of nitrous oxide during the preparation of gingival cavities for porcelain inlays. Parenthetically, it is appropriate that such interest should be developed at the University, for Iowa was perhaps the first state university to provide in its teaching hospitals a formal residency program in general anesthesia for physicians.[10] A well-known advocate of nitrous oxide, Clements,[9] in 1945 wrote that "analgesia is now widely used and its value in the dental field firmly established." His short description of sedation is excellent. In 1956 Henning Ruben, of Copenhagen, published in Danish a classic monograph on universal analgesia (sedation),[26] which unfortunately was not translated. Currently the English-language text of Langa[20] enjoys wide circulation.

ETHER

William T. G. Morton was a former pupil and partner of Horace Wells. He realized that inhalation anesthesia would rapidly build a dental practice. Morton acted upon the advice of C. T. Jackson, a chemist and physician, and substituted ether for nitrous oxide. Thus it was that on the morning of October 18, 1846, a dentist once again stood before the medical students of John C. Warren to demonstrate anesthesia.

The apparatus available for administering gas anesthetics was a bag for nitrous oxide and a modified hollow glass ball with an inhalation mouthpiece reminiscent of that on a skin diver's snorkel. Poor Wells in his demonstration before the students of John Warren had the responsibility of acting as both anesthetist and surgeon. The more fortunate Morton administered ether to a receptive patient while Warren performed the surgery. John Warren is today honored because he had the objectivity to realize that surgical anesthesia was a reality.

Morton tried to patent "Letheon," as he termed his compound of ether. Further, he entered vigorously into the controversy concerning the priority of the discovery of anestheisa. For some years he was lionized, and during the early part of this period Oliver Wendell Holmes suggested the name of "anesthesia" for the state produced and of "anesthetic" for the stupefying compound. Morton was the first specialist in the adminstration of anesthetics and the first manufacturer of anesthetic equipment.[2]

The first physician to limit his practice to anesthesia was John Snow. His genius and ability contributed largely to the advancement of anesthesiology as it progressed "from the empirical application of a single observation to a discipline of medicine based solidly on scientific experimentation."[3] Snow was the first to classify the signs of ether anesthesia into a clinically useful sequence. He conducted a scientific series of physical and physiological experiments on laboratory animals and on himself. His first human subjects were outpatients requiring dental extractions at St. George's Hospital, and on January 28, 1847, six weeks after the first use of ether in England, Snow started his specialty of administering ether for major surgery. In a short time all the ether practice of London was in his hands. Later he twice administered chloroform to Queen Victoria, during the births of Prince Leopold and Princess Beatrice. The first of these administrations had great significance for the acceptance of anesthesia, as we shall later see.

CHLOROFORM

Sir James Y. Simpson, a Scot, introduced ether into obstetrical practice on January 19, 1847. He found the odor disagreeable and in his search for an alternative introduced chloroform to clinical practice. Three men—Wells, Morton and Simpson—had three different motives and employed three different gases, the clinical applications of which within three years burst with explosive suddenness upon the medical and dental professions.

Austin C. Hewitt, hearing of Simpson's progress, reportedly imported at a fabulous price a small quantity of chloroform. The result was that he may have been the first man in the United States to use the drug, and was certainly the first to advocate the performance of surgical operations in a state of chloroform *analgesia.* Hewitt later closed his medical and surgical practice to open a dental office in the city of Chicago. In 1893 and 1895 he read before the Iowa State Dental Society papers on chloroform analgesia "which so impressed the Society that a committee was appointed to visit Dr. Hewitt at his office in Chicago and make a report of what he was doing."[12] The committee had sent, prior to their visit, a list of procedures they wished to see performed with the aid of chloroform analgesia. The list covered the entire field of the general practice of dentistry and the committee, with DeFord as chairman, submitted to the Society a very favorable report; it included the recommendation that a chair of anesthesia be established in every dental school so that local and general anesthetics might be scientifically studied and taught. It concluded that the dental profession at large, as well as the Iowa State Dental Society, owed Dr. Hewitt a debt of gratitude for making public his discoveries. Hewitt stated: "That in all the range of operative dentistry and in the demands of oral surgery, there are but four to six operations demanding its exhibition to complete anesthesia. The obtundent influence is ample. Under no circumstances is a dentist justified in fully anesthetizing a patient for extraction of teeth, for minor operations, or for oral surgery. During a somewhat lengthened practice, never an accident or an approach to an accident has occurred."

"As a result of careful study and extensive use, Dr. Hewitt does not hesitate to commend its general use as an *obtundent.*" When administered by Hewitt's method, chloroform produced no apparent untoward reactions; he felt that it was "a substance in the hands of the unskilled and reckless, as dangerous to human life as prussic acid or dynamite, but used properly, legitimately, as safe as the odor from the heart of a rose."[12] DeFord also recognized the critical role of the anesthetist, and in the chapter "Relative Safety of General Anesthetics" often referred to the principle of responsibility embodied in Hewitt's colorful summary.

CONTROVERSY

When Simpson introduced chloroform for childbirth a significant controvery arose. The clergy spoke from a traditional misconception of God; in essence their argument was that God ordained the pain of childbirth. Simpson was a worthy opponent, well equipped for the battle. Still, although scientists pride themselves on the irrefutable logic of their objective conclusions, it was the choice of a woman who set the "fashion." When John Snow administered an anesthetic to Queen Victoria for the birth of Prince Leopold, to which we previously alluded, the administration did more than provide freedom from pain; it more effectively promoted the acceptance of anesthesia than did the logical position of anesthesia's two great champions, Simpson and Boston's

Channing.[2] As an example of the widespread lay interest in the application of anesthesia we may read a letter from President Tyler written to Dr. J. K. Mitchell requesting that Dr. Mitchell forward a bottle of ether with instructions concerning "the precise mode of the use of ether in cases of childbirth." The President was anticipating a birth in his own family.[31]

The dental profession was reluctant to accept the great advance, which in its early stages was probably more like analgesia than anesthesia as known today. There were several apparent reasons. Mountebanks and charlatans abounded, and some abused the use of the gases to prey on the public. Dental surgeons and the public press decried such practices. An alarming number of deaths occurred during the administration of anesthetics for dental extractions as well as for general surgery. Archer[2] cites in part the official statement of the American Society of Dental Surgeons regarding ether and chloroform in dentistry "... Hence, in all minor operations in surgery their administration is forbidden; and that their demand in the practice of dental surgery is small ..." Harris, Westcott, and Dwinnell declared themselves less than enthusiastic about the administration of sulfuric ether to extract teeth.

In England, as reported by Thomas,[29] Fowell and Tomes cited the pro's, con's and reasoned hesitation. Fowell in his *Treatise on Dentistry* (1859) said "Some persons, I am sorry to say, have become so enamored of chloroform or ether ... as to refuse to permit the operation (of dental extraction) without its assistance ... but when it comes to the removal of a tooth, which is an act simple in its execution and quick in its effect, I must confess that I think it is indiscreet ..." The great dental surgeon John Tomes, who delivered the most comprehensive early essay upon the use of anesthesia in dental operations, summarized, "We surely use a great power to overcome a very trifling difficulty, when we give chloroform preparatory to extracting an ordinary tooth." He was also aware that what we call analgesia was oftentimes sufficient: "On many occasions the patient has been perfectly aware of the steps of the operation, has felt the instrument grasp the tooth ... and yet has felt little or no pain."

Until 1884 it was just too bad for the individual who required eye surgery, a dental extraction, the removal of an ingrown toenail, or a minor operation. During the Civil War when more than 80,000 general anesthetics were administered there were *reported* at least 256 major operations without anesthesia.[32] The reason was simple. The patient and the doctor often concluded that the pain of the procedure was less noxious than the after-effects of the anesthetic. The available apparatus and techniques of administration limited the use of anesthetics to the most urgent cases. Obviously something was needed to abolish fear or pain in dentistry and minor surgery, and especially in eye surgery where general anesthesia was contraindicated because of the after-effects.

LOCAL ANESTHESIA

Cocaine

In Vienna General Hospital two young medical men, Carl Köller and Sigmund Freud, were investigating the psychic effect of cocaine. Cocaine had been extracted from the leaves of the coca shrub of South America in 1860 by the chemist Niemann, who reported that "it produced temporary insensibility on the part of the tongue with which it came in contact."[21] Strangely, the report did not give Köller a clue to the local anesthetic effect of cocaine. Freud had obtained a little of the limited amount of available cocaine; in order to test its effect both he and Köller took some. Freud soon left on a vacation and then Köller suddenly remembered three important things: (1) that he was searching for something to numb the eye, (2) that the cocaine he and Freud had swallowed made their tongues numb, and (3) that Freud had left him a small amount. Köller prepared a solution of cocaine in water and tested it in the eye of a frog, the eye of a guinea pig, and in his own eye. The result was numbness of the eye. Such was the discovery of local anesthesia. Raper[24] and Thorwald[30] give an interesting account of this event and the paper Köller wrote about his discovery which a colleague read to members of the German Ophthalmological Society at Heidelberg on September 15, 1884.

The Syringe

Shortly after Köller's publication, William Halstead, a New York surgeon, started injecting cocaine near nerve trunks blocking the region supplied by that nerve. He employed an adaptation of the hollow needle hypodermic syringe which Wood and Pravaz had perfected in 1853 for the purpose of injecting morphine for the relief of neuralgic pain in a patient's shoulder. The perfection of a functional syringe was an important step in the achievement of local anesthesia.[7]

Nerve Blocks

By September 1885 Halstead, and his associate Hall who may have been the first man to report the block of the inferior alveolar nerve,[16] had employed cocaine in over 1000 cases. Many individuals were administering the drug and within $3\frac{1}{2}$ months following its discovery American and Canadian investigators had published some 60 papers on the subject—in dentistry and in practically every practice of medicine.[24] Raymond[25] reports that after Halstead administered an inferior alveolar nerve block to a patient with a hypersensitive tooth, the tooth was prepared for a restoration without discomfort.

It was soon found, however, that cocaine was far from an ideal anesthetic. It is a dangerous drug capable of effects ranging from local gangrene to systemic, sometimes fatal, toxicity, and to possible addiction. Immediately investigators sought to enhance its good properties and modify or eliminate its hazards.

In 1900 Braun mixed an extract of the adrenals of animals with a cocaine solution and injected the mixture into his forearm. "He realized at once that a new era for local anesthesia had arrived."[7] In 1903 he published his ingenious experiments with a cocaine-epinephrine solution. The technique of local anesthesia was simplified because the vasoconstrictor limits the absorption of the local anesthetic, thereby decreasing systemic toxicity. It also prolongs the duration of anesthesia, decreases the amount of the drug needed and lessens hemorrhage from surgical procedures in the area.

Novocain

The appearance of Novocain, synthesized by Einhorn in 1905, made local anesthesia a reality upon which advances in surgery could be built, and the use of the anesthetic block in diagnosis, prognosis, and therapy could be established.[5,15] Novocain is still a reliable and standard product but is superseded by lidocaine and mepivacaine hydrochloride in dentistry.

Nerve Blocks: Clinical Applications

However, nerve blocks for major surgery almost floundered until it was firmly established that "Anatomy is the foundation on which the edifice of regional anesthesia is built."[19,27]

The first surgeons, who administered their own anesthetic solutions, infiltrating ahead of the area of incision as the need arose, realized that the need for a knowledge of regional and topographic anatomy, especially with regard to nerve distribution, is beyond discussion. Further, this particular study of anatomy must be approached from an angle previously unknown to medical students and unfamiliar to surgeons. In 1914 Dr. Guido Fischer, a German dentist, was brought to the United States to teach for the first time the now accepted technique of block anesthesia. Still, Smith in his entirely new text of dental anesthesia (1920) stated that the majority of dentists were not practicing nerve blocks but were simply making subperiosteal or submucous injections as had been practiced almost since the time that cocaine was first injected. He concluded: "The fundamental basis of nerve blocking is not only a thorough knowledge of nervous anatomy, but also of the surrounding anatomic structures"[27] and judged that the mastery of anatomy combined with other aspects of technique would make nerve blocking a pleasure to any operator.

Of more than parenthetical interest to dentists is the observation that it may have been Smith's monumental text that inspired that great protagonist of spinal anesthesia, Pitkin, to share his own knowledge by publishing *Conduction Anesthesia.*[23] The first chapter of the book demonstrates how mistaken but "Inherited Concepts Concerning Conduction Anesthesia" are perpetuated. It is illuminating reading, particularly for those inclined to evade the discipline of a review of anatomy.

In the blocking of the fifth nerve the dentist draws upon the anatomical descriptions of, among others, Galen from the second century, Fallopio (1532–62), Meckel's description of the nerve and the pterygopalatine (Meckel's) ganglion, and Bell's demonstration in 1829 that the fifth cranial nerve is sensorimotor. The delicacy of Bell's[4] drawings in the Philosophical Transactions of the Royal Society of London are not to be exceeded (see page 112).

In spite of the available descriptive material most dentists did not have the ability to administer local anesthetics in 1927. So the company now known as Cook-Waite organized a professional division, staffed it with skilled, qualified dentists, and assigned them as rapidly as possible to teach block anesthesia to as many dentists as possible. Within a few years more than 15,000 dentists had attended the clinics. These practitioners, combined with those contemporaneously graduating from dental schools, brought acceptance of the local anesthetic techniques to the United States.

The next steps were in the areas of improving methods of administering the gaseous anesthetics, discovering new inhalation anesthetics, and, of course, the introduction of intravenous anesthesia.

In the late 1860s Colton had popularized nitrous oxide for dental extractions in his "Dental Institutes." The gas was supplied in rubber bags in quantities sufficient for one or two patients, a drawback to transport and storage which Thomas Evans circumvented by liquefying the gas and confining it to small iron containers. It was Evans who, against formidable opposition, introduced nitrous oxide anesthesia to England and the continent. Then the physiologist Paul Bert, in France, and the surgeon Edmund Andrews, in Chicago, added oxygen to the mixture to make it suitable for major surgery. Still it required an additional 30 years before Frederick W. Hewitt, more than any other, made nitrous oxide-oxygen anesthesia practical.

ETHYL CHLORIDE

Two dentists introduced ethyl chloride into clinical practice about 1895, although Flourens in 1851 as well as John Snow rejected it as a respiratory anesthetic. Carlson of Gothenburg and Thiesing of Hildesheim both noticed that the vapors of ethyl chloride spray, used to "freeze" the gums, caused sleep when inhaled. They followed the observation with animal and human laboratory experimentation.[2,24] Jacobs and Gobie, working at Forsyth Dental Infirmary, introduced the technique which made ethyl chloride a familiar name to American dentistry. Booth has recorded its manner of use at the clinic.[6] That Forsyth was a prime user of ethyl chloride can be seen from the clinical records—632 administrations in 1915, climbing to a high of 26,211 in 1928 and then decreasing to the point of discontinuation in 1955 when it was supplanted by nitrous oxide-oxygen, supplemented when necessary with Vinethene, and wherever possible accompanied by infiltration of lidocaine.[28]

GAS MACHINES

Charles K. Teter, a dentist of Cleveland, brought out the second machine for the administration of nitrous oxide and oxygen in 1902. E. I. McKesson, M.D., an associate professor of physiological chemistry at Toledo Medical College, became interested in anesthesia and in 1910 perfected the first "intermittent flow" machine with accurate percentage control for the two gases. In the meantime Heidbrink, still remembering the torture of having impacted mandibular molars removed without anesthesia as a dental student, experimented with the Teter machine and finally built an entirely new machine in 1908. These three, Teter, McKesson and Heidbrink, through articles, lectures, and clinical demonstrations were largely responsible for bringing about the use of nitrous oxide in major surgery in the United States.[2]

ETHYLENE, CYCLOPROPANE, AND DIVINYL ETHER

Between 1920 and 1933 three important anesthetics were introduced—ethylene, cyclopropane, and divinyl ether. Archer reports: "The first dental extractions under ethylene and oxygen anesthesia, numbering approximately 100 cases, were performed by Charles Dodd at the Salvation Army Clinic in Chicago with Luckhart supervising the anesthetics."[2] On November 6, 1933, Thomas Cook, at the Hospital of the University of Pennsylvania, performed the first dental operation with the patient anesthetized with Vinethene—the trade name, so well known to dentists, of divinyl ether.[2,24]

BARBITURATES

The stage was set for the intravenous anesthetics when Fischer and Von Mering introduced barbital (Veronal) into medicine in 1903. Veronal is still one of the best hypnotics.[15] Fischer received the Nobel Prize in recognition of his splendid achievement. Lundy later thoroughly investigated a barbituric acid derivative at the Mayo Clinic, and in American dentistry that drug, Pentothal, is a standby for intravenous anesthesia.[24] At about the same time a London dentist, S. L. Drummond-Jackson, pioneered in the use of intravenous barbiturate anesthesia (hexobarbital) to accomplish both restorative dentistry and oral surgery,[13,14] while many dentists in England and Europe employed intravenous anesthesia for oral surgery. Adrian Hubbell studied with Lundy at the Mayo Clinic (1937–40) and was, with Wyckoff[33] and Bullard,[8] a pioneer in the use of intravenous anesthesia for ambulatory oral surgery patients. Hubbell[17] was the first North American to adopt in his office the routine full-scale administration of intravenous anesthesia without premedication as the sole agent for ambulatory patients having oral operations. In 1945, Jorgensen[18] was one of the first to refine the intravenous administration of barbiturates, soon combined with analgesics, to the point that he could routinely determine precisely the desired stage of light sedation for "problem" dental patients. After obtaining light sedation he administered nerve blocks to provide the necessary local anesthesia. Interestingly enough, routine intravenous anesthesia and sedation for the ambulatory dental patiant in private offices seems to be a unique contribution of southern Californians to their North American dental colleagues and patients.

NEUROLEPTIC-NARCOTIC COMBINATIONS

Recently much attention has been directed to states known either as "neuroleptic analgesia" or dissociative anesthesia. In the former instance, the patient is quiescent and quite indifferent to environmental stimuli, although not asleep. In the latter, the patient, during induction, feels dissociated not only from his environment but from his extremities. The two drugs most often associated with these states are, respectively, Innovar (fentanyl-droperidol) and Ketamine (cyclohexylamine).[15] Although not yet adaptable to routine use in dental offices, these drugs lend encouragement as the search for the "ideal" drug continues.

EPILOGUE

A little over a hundred years of progress in dental anesthesia has not added much veneer to the specter of fear and pain portrayed in Szekely's characterization of the modern dentist (Fig. 2–1). That is strange, for the predecessors and contemporaries of today's dentist have given him inexpensive, readily available, reliable and invincible weapons with which to vanquish fear and pain. We know where we have been. Where do we go?

BIBLIOGRAPHY

1. Archer, W. H.: Life and letters of Horace Wells, discoverer of anesthesia. J. Amer. Coll. Dent. *11*:81, 1944.
2. Archer, W. H.: *A Manual of Dental Anesthesia.* Philadelphia, W. B. Saunders Co., 1952, pp. 1–34.
3. Bergman, N. A.: The legacy of John Snow. Anesthesiology *19*:595, 1958.
4. Bell, Charles: On the nerves of the face, being a second paper on that subject. Philos. Trans. Roy. Soc. London, 1829, pp. 317–330.
5. Bonica, J. J.: *The Management of Pain.* Philadelphia, Lea & Febiger, 1953, pp. 17–24.
6. Booth, N. A.: Ethyl chloride: Its use at the Forsyth Dental Infirmary for Children. Oral Surg. *3*:1260, 1950.
7. Braun, Heinrich, and Harris, M. L. (translator): *Local Anesthesia, Its Scientific Basis and Practical Use*, 2nd Amer. ed. Philadelphia, Lea & Febiger, 1924.
8. Bullard, O. K.: Intravenous anesthesia in office practice for operations in exodontia and oral surgery; based on an experience of 946 cases. Anesth. Analg. *19*:26, 1940.
9. Clements, F. W.: *Nitrous Oxide-Oxygen Anesthesia.* Philadelphia, Lea & Febiger, 1945, pp. 270–273.
10. Davis, D. A. and Moyers, Jack: Harding of Iowa. In *Clinical Anesthesia, Historical Vignettes of Anesthesia* (Davis, D. A., ed.). Philadelphia, F. A. Davis Co., 1968, p. 68.
11. Deaderick, W. H.: Case of removal of a portion of the lower maxillary bone. Amer. Med. Rec. *6*:516, 1823.
12. DeFord, W. H.: *Lectures on General Anesthetics in Dentistry.* Kansas City, John T. Nolde Mfg. Co., 1908, Chaps. 8 and 19.
13. Drummond-Jackson, S. L.: Evipal anaesthesia in dentistry. Dent. Cosmos *77*:130, 1935.
14. Drummond-Jackson, S. L.: A milestone in intravenous anesthesia. Corresp. Brit. Dent. J. *113*:404, 1962.
15. Goodman, L. S., and Gilman, Alfred: *The Pharmacological Basis of Therapeutics*, 4th ed. New York, The Macmillan Co., 1970.
16. Hall, R. J.: Hydrochlorate of cocaine. Corresp. N. Y. Med. J. *40*:643, 1884.
17. Hubbell, A. O. and Adams, R. C.: Intravenous anesthesia for dental surgery with sodium ethyl (1-methylbutyl) thiobarbituric acid. J. Amer. Dent. Assoc. *27*:1186, 1940.
18. Jorgensen, N. B., and Leffingwell, F. E.: Premedication in dentistry. J. Southern Calif. Dent. Assoc. *21*:1, 1953.
19. Labat, Gaston. *Regional Anesthesia*, 2nd ed. Philadelphia, W. B. Saunders Co., 1928.
20. Langa, Harry: *Relative Analgesia in Dental Practice. Inhalation Analgesia with Nitrous Oxide.* Philadelphia, W. B. Saunders Co., 1968.
21. Martindale, William: *Coca, Cocaine and its Salts.* London, H. K. Lewis & Co., Ltd., 1886.
22. McDowell, Frank, and Ohlwiler, David: Collective review. Mandibular resection and replacement. Int. Abstr. Surg. *115*:103, 1962.
23. Pitkin, G. B.: *Conduction Anesthesia*, 2nd ed. Philadelphia, J. B. Lippincott Co., 1953.
24. Raper, H. R.: *Man against Pain.* New York, Prentice-Hall, Inc., 1945.
25. Raymond, E. H.: Hydrochlorate of cocaine as a local anesthetic in dental surgery. Dent. Cosmos *27*:207, 1885.
26. Ruben, Henning: *Grundlag for Universel Analgesi.* København, Dansk Tandlaegeforening, 1958. (*Basis for Universal Analgesia.* Copenhagen, Danish Dental Society, 1958.)
27. Smith, A. E.: *Block Anesthesia and Allied Subjects.* St. Louis, C. V. Mosby Co., 1920.
28. Springer, James, and Saglio, Diane: Personal communication. Boston, Forsyth Dental Center, Oct. 26, 1965.
29. Thomas, K. B.: Some early papers on dental anaesthesia. Brit. Dent. J. *116*:139, 1964.
30. Thorwald, Jurgen, and Winston, Richard and Clara (translators): *The Triumph of Surgery.* New York, Pantheon Books, Inc., p. 280.
31. Tyler, John: Letter No. 4969. Birmingham. Lawrence Reynolds Library, University of Alabama.
32. U. S. Surgeon General's Office. *The Medical and Surgical History of the War of the Rebellion* (1861–5). Washington, Government Printing Office, 1883, 2 vols. Vol 2, prt. 3, pp. 887–98.
33. Wyckoff, B. S.: Intravenous anesthesia in oral surgery. Amer. J. Orthodont. *24*:875, 1938.

Appendix

COMMONLY USED DRUGS

Drug — Generic Name	*Drug* — Trade Name	*Suggested Supply; Injectable (Sterile Water May Be Required) Unless Oral Administration Noted*	*Manufacturer*
1. Aminophylline U.S.P.	Aminophyllin	250 mg/10 ml ampule	Scarl & Co., G.O. P.O. Box 5110, Chicago, Illinois 60680
2. Atropine sulfate U.S.P.	Ampoule atropine sulfate Atropine sulfate tablets	0.4 mg/ml, oral 1/100 gr 1/50 gr, 1/200 gr	Eli Lilly & Company, Indianapolis, Indiana 46206
3. Dexamethasone sodium phosphate U.S.P.	Decadron phosphate	4 mg/ml in 1- or 5-ml vials	Merck, Sharp & Dohme, West Point, Pennsylvania 19486
4. Diazepam N.F.	Valium	5 mg/ml in 2-ml ampules	Roche Laboratories, Nutley, New Jersey 07110
5. Diphenhydramine hydrochloride U.S.P.	Benadryl	1-ml ampules, 50 mg/ml	Parke, Davis & Company, Detroit, Michigan 48232
6. Epinephrine U.S.P.	Adrenalin chloride solution Suprarenin; Epinephrine	1:1,000 (1 mg/ml) 30-ml vials	Parke, Davis & Company, Detroit, Michigan 48232
7. Meperidine hydrochloride	Demerol hydrochloride	50-mg/ml ampules, vials	Winthrop Laboratories, 90 Park Ave., New York, N. Y. 10016
8. Mephentermine sulfate	Wyamine sulfate	15 mg/ml vials of 1 ml	Wyeth Laboratories, P.O. Box 8299, Philadelphia, Pa. 19101

9.	Methohexital sodium	Brevital sodium	500-mg, 2.5-gm, 5.0-gm ampules	Eli Lilly & Company, Indianapolis, Indiana 46206
10.	Pentobarbital sodium U.S.P.	Nembutal sodium	50 mg/ml in 2-ml ampules or 20-ml vials	Abbott Laboratories, North Chicago, Illinois 60064
11.	Pentylenetetrazol	Metrazol	100-mg/ml ampules	Knoll Pharmaceutical, Orange, New Jersey 07501
12.	Phenylephrine hydrochloride, U.S.P.	Neo-Synephrine hydrochloride; Phenylephrine hydrochloride	10 mg/ml in 1-ml ampules or 5-ml vials	Winthrop Laboratories, 90 Park Ave., New York, N. Y. 10016
13.	Prochlorperazine edisylate U.S.P.	Compazine	5-mg/ml ampules or multiple-dose vials	Smith, Kline & French Lab., 1500 Spring Garden St., Philadelphia, Pa. 19101
14.	Scopolamine hydrobromide U.S.P.		0.32-mg/ml ampules	Burroughs Wellcome & Co. (USA) Inc., Tuckahoe, N. Y. 10707
15.	Secobarbital sodium U.S.P.	Seconal sodium	Capsules 0.0325 gm, 0.05 gm, and 0.1 gm	Eli Lilly & Company, Indianapolis, Indiana 46206
16.	Sterile water for injection U.S.P.		Vials	Cutter Laboratories, Berkeley, California 94710
17.	Succinylcholine chloride U.S.P.	Anectine	20-mg/ml vials (10 ml)	Burroughs Wellcome & Co. (U.S.A.) Inc., Tuckahoe, N. Y. 10707
18.	Thiopental sodium U.S.P.	Pentothal sodium	Available in sizes from: 500-mg ampules to 10-gm/500 ml multiple-dose containers	Abbott Laboratories, North Chicago, Ill. 60064

Index

Italic page number indicates an illustration